ALLEN CARR'S
EASY WAY
FOR WOMEN TO
QUIT
DRINKING

SIRIUS

To Cris Hay—Allen Carr's Easyway to Stop Drinking Alcohol Therapist Extraordinaire

SIRIUS

This edition published in 2024 by Sirius Publishing, a division of
Arcturus Publishing Limited,
26/27 Bickels Yard, 151–153 Bermondsey Street,
London SE1 3HA

ISBN: 978-1-78599-147-9
AD004833US

Printed in the UK

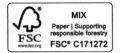

ALLEN CARR

Allen Carr was a chain-smoker for over 30 years. In 1983, after countless failed attempts to quit, he went from 100 cigarettes a day to zero without suffering withdrawal pangs, without using willpower, and without putting on weight. He realized that he had discovered what the world had been waiting for—the easy way to stop smoking—and embarked on a mission to help cure the world's smokers.

As a result of the phenomenal success of his method, he gained an international reputation as the world's leading expert on quitting smoking and his network of centers now spans the globe. His first book, *Allen Carr's Easy Way to Stop Smoking*, has sold over 15 million copies, remains a global bestseller, and has been published in over 40 different languages. Hundreds of thousands of smokers have successfully quit at Allen Carr's Easyway Centers where, with a success rate of over 90 percent, they guarantee you'll find it easy to quit or your money back.

Allen Carr's Easyway method has been successfully applied to a host of issues including weight control, alcohol, and other addictions and fears. A list of Allen Carr centers appears at the back of this book. Should you require any assistance or if you have any questions, please do not hesitate to contact your nearest center.

For more information about Allen Carr's Easyway, please visit

www.allencarr.com

Allen Carr's Easyway

The key that will set you free

CONTENTS

PREFACE

By Colleen Dwyer, Senior Therapist, Allen Carr's Easyway

I stopped drinking in July 1997 at Allen Carr's center in Raynes Park, London. Having started at 13, I had an extraordinary capacity for alcohol and I quickly sank into the alcohol trap. By the age of 27, I was an out-and-out alcoholic. Booze came before friends, before family, before work, and before my own desire to stop. I remember feeling so nervous and uncertain on my arrival at the center, but, sure enough, by the end of that six-hour seminar I was mentally prepared for the change.

Allen Carr's Easyway had completely reframed the entire issue of drinking in my mind. I hadn't yet tested out my new way of thinking, but I already knew I had no regrets about stopping and I was certain that I could do it. Those six hours completely changed my life. I dread to think what would have become of me if I had continued to drink and, although I knew I'd made the right decision by stopping, I didn't quite understand the impact it would have on my future life.

Regaining my confidence and self-respect was nothing less than wonderful. I was almost like a child experiencing situations for the first time: my first dinner out with friends where I didn't drink, my first visit to a bar and not drinking, first birthday, first vacation, first Christmas, even my first crisis situation that I took in my stride—without alcohol. I approached them all with a sense of curiosity rather than one of foreboding. And as I found my feet and became more and more certain that life without alcohol wasn't just a nice idea on paper but a truly fantastic reality, I was walking on air.

Nights that were once lost to wine, embarrassing encounters and endless boring debates about nothing turned into nights worth remembering, spent with family and friends, doing a whole number of different and enjoyable activities. And I rediscovered the pleasure of waking up in the morning feeling fresh and happy, not guilty and hungover. I lost weight, I looked a lot better, I became productive and constructive, and I began to like myself again.

I will always be grateful to Allen Carr for sharing his amazing method with the world and I was delighted to be given the opportunity to work for Easyway and help other people to escape the alcohol trap as I did. Allen originally devised his method to help people quit smoking and it was—and still is—a phenomenal success. More than 400,000 people have attended Easyway centers in over 50 countries and Allen Carr's Easyway books have been translated into over 40 languages, have sold more than 20 million copies, and have been read by an estimated 30 to 40 million people. This success has been achieved not through advertising or marketing but through the personal recommendations of the millions of people who have succeeded with the method. Allen Carr's Easyway has spread all over the world for one reason alone: BECAUSE IT WORKS.

As I discovered to my eternal gratitude, it doesn't just work for smoking. It has been applied successfully to alcohol, weight, gambling, and even debt. *The Easy Way for Women to Quit Drinking* presents the method to women who, like me all those years ago, are suffering the misery and stigma of being a woman with a drink problem and are desperate to find a way out of the trap.

I haven't touched alcohol since that visit to Allen Carr's London Center in 1997. I have no desire to. I feel happy and healthy in a way I simply could not imagine when I was drinking. I have no doubt whatsoever that the method laid out in this book will help you change your life just as it changed mine. All you have to do is follow the instructions.

INTRODUCTION

By John Dicey, Global CEO & Senior Therapist, Allen Carr's Easyway

For a third of a century Allen Carr chain-smoked 60 to 100 cigarettes a day. With the exception of acupuncture, he'd tried all the conventional and unconventional methods to quit without success.

As he describes it: "It was like being between the devil and the deep blue sea. I desperately wanted to quit, but whenever I tried I was utterly miserable.

"No matter how long I survived without a cigarette, I never felt completely free. It was as if I had lost my best friend, my crutch, my character, my very personality. In those days I believed there were such types as addictive personalities or confirmed smokers, and because my family were all heavy smokers, I believed that there was something in our genes that meant we couldn't enjoy life or cope with stress without smoking."

Eventually he gave up even trying to quit, believing: once a smoker, always a smoker. Then he discovered something which motivated him to try again.

"I went overnight from 100 cigarettes a day to zero—without any bad temper or sense of loss, void, or depression. On the contrary, I actually enjoyed the process. I knew I was already a nonsmoker even before I had extinguished my final cigarette and I've never had the slightest urge to smoke since."

It didn't take Allen long to realize that he had discovered a method of quitting that would enable any smoker to quit:

- EASILY, IMMEDIATELY,. AND PERMANENTLY

- WITHOUT USING WILLPOWER, AIDS, SUBSTITUTES, OR GIMMICKS

- WITHOUT SUFFERING DEPRESSION OR WITHDRAWAL SYMPTOMS

- WITHOUT GAINING WEIGHT

After using his smoking friends and relatives as guinea pigs, he gave up his lucrative profession as a qualified accountant and set up a center to help other smokers to quit.

He called his method "EASYWAY" and so successful has it been that there are now Allen Carr's Easyway centers in more than 150 cities in 50 countries worldwide. Bestselling books based on his method are now translated into over 40 languages, with more being added each year.

It quickly became clear to Allen that his method could be applied to any drug. The method has helped tens of millions of people quit smoking, alcohol, and other drugs, as well as to stop gambling, stop overeating, and stop overspending.

The method works by unraveling the misconceptions that make people believe that they get some benefit from the very thing that's harming them.

This book applies the method to the issue of alcohol and unlike other methods it does not require willpower.

Too good to be true? All you have to do is read the book in its entirety, follow all the instructions, and you cannot fail.

I'm aware that the claims of the method's success might appear far-fetched or exaggerated, at times even outrageous. That was certainly my reaction when I first heard them. I was incredibly fortunate to attend Allen Carr's center in London in 1997—yet I did so under duress. I had agreed to go, at the request of my wife, on the understanding that when I walked out of the center and remained a smoker she would leave it at least 12 months before hassling me about stopping smoking again. No one was more surprised than me, or perhaps my wife, that Allen Carr's Easyway method set me free from my 80-a-day addiction.

I was so inspired that I hassled and harangued Allen Carr and Robin Hayley (now chairman of Allen Carr's Easyway) to let me get involved in their quest to cure the world of smoking. I was incredibly fortunate to have succeeded in convincing them to allow me to do so. Being trained by Allen Carr and Robin Hayley was one of the most rewarding experiences of my life. To be able to count Allen as not only my coach and mentor but also my friend was an amazing honor and privilege. Allen Carr and Robin Hayley trained me well: I personally went on to treat more than 30,000 smokers at Allen's original London center, and became part of the team that has taken Allen's method from Berlin to Bogota, from New Zealand to New York, from Sydney to Santiago. Tasked by Allen with ensuring that his legacy achieves its full potential, we've taken Allen Carr's Easyway from videos to DVD, from centers to apps, from computer games to audio books, to online programs and beyond. We've a long way to go, with so many addictions and issues to apply the method to, and this book plays a special part in our quest.

The honor of adding a light editorial touch to update and develop Allen's method in this book has fallen to me and the amazing Colleen Dwyer, one of the most senior Allen Carr's Easyway therapists in the world.

Editing Allen's work as we have enables us to apply the most up-to-date, cutting-edge version of his method to a whole host of issues, while inserting, where necessary, up-to-date examples and references within the text.

Follow Allen Carr's instructions and you'll find it not only easy to be free from alcohol, but you'll actually enjoy the whole process of quitting. You won't just be free; you'll be happy to be free. That might sound too good to be true at the moment, but read on: You have nothing to lose and absolutely everything to gain. Let me pass you into the safest of hands—over to Allen Carr.

Chapter 1

WOMEN AND ALCOHOL

A woman with a drink problem gets very little sympathy from society. It's time you stopped suffering and got the help you need to escape from the alcohol trap.

Since I wrote my first book, *The Easy Way to Stop Smoking*, in 1985 I've learned something new about addiction practically every day. Over the years I've incorporated this knowledge into revised editions of my books. Up until my first book that covered addiction specifically from a female angle, *The Easy Way for Women to Quit Smoking*, everything I wrote was from my perspective. In this book, like the others that I've subsequently written exclusively for women, I have tried to let my perceptions take a backseat to allow the experiences and insights of women who have escaped to freedom by using my method to speak through me. The majority of clients who attend my centers throughout the world are women, so it seems appropriate, when possible, to produce versions of Easyway devoted to them. Or is it?

I've been asked frequently if it is necessary—or even politically correct—to write specifically about women and drinking. It's important to appreciate that my method works for all drinkers regardless of their gender, so what is the point in women-specific versions of the method? From my own experiences, as well as those of senior therapists at my centers, there are recurring issues regarding stopping drinking which often only apply to women. We are able to address these at our live center sessions; it is part of the skill of being one of my therapist team. Whether male or female, their success rates are equal regardless of the gender of the clients.

Now, in the *Easy Way for Women to Quit Drinking*, I want to show a wider audience how the method can be as successful at dealing with these very specific anxieties as it is with the broad spectrum of obstacles to stopping drinking.

Are men and women so different? Yes and no. But one thing is certainly true: Some women drinkers suffer a far greater fear of stopping drinking than men. We know this from concerns that they raise at our center sessions. It's certainly not a case of men being too shy to make their fears known—simply that men generally do not share the anxieties that women frequently describe.

Drinking can appear to be part of a woman's support network. Whether it's a drink in a bar after work, or a drink while cooking dinner, or a drink after putting the kids to bed, or even all three, drink appears to be an integral part of her life, and inextricably linked to the image she has of herself. The thought of losing a part of her support mechanism or stress safety valve is terrifying to a woman drinker, even if, on the face of it, she is the most accomplished multirole performer.

The "special relationship" that women have with alcohol is intrinsically linked with how and why women function in the way that they do and with their differently acquired views of how to deal with life.

The drinks industry understands this very well. Not only do they understand it, they manipulate it mercilessly. At what point did a glass of wine in a bar cease to be a normal measure (around a sixth of a bottle) and begin to be served in *Regular* (still bigger than the old norm) or *Large*—at times resembling a bucket of wine rather than a glass? The answer is that deals have been designed to encourage the purchase of a whole bottle rather than just a few glasses. Aside from changes in pub/bar culture, the drinks industry as a whole has spent, and continues to spend, huge sums of money on the psychological profiling of women. They are doing their best to get inside the heads of women, to understand how they see things, how they think, and the ways in which their psychology differs from men.

The basic truths of the alcohol trap will never change—basic truths that Easyway addresses so successfully. The ways in which women fall into that trap have changed, however, and women who want to escape must be made aware of those ways if they are to succeed in avoiding the trap permanently.

The alcohol industry has had a huge hand in this change to the way women drink, but so too has social change and, by extension, women themselves. The social revolution begun in the 1960s has bred a cash cow for the drinks industry, a lucrative new market, especially among what it refers to as YAFs (Young Adult Females). It is a tragic irony that in becoming liberated in one sense women should be colluding in their enslavement in another.

One thing is certain: Once you see the alcohol trap in its true light, you will achieve true liberation and you will know this really is the easy way. But whichever way you look at it, women are drinking more than they used to.

In the U.S.A., from the early 1990s to the early 2000s, the percentage of women who classified themselves as drinkers spiked: Among white women it was up 24 percent; hispanic women 33 percent; black women 42 percent. By 2010, Gallup reported that over two-thirds of U.S. women drank regularly and that it was the better-educated, more affluent women who were drinking the most.

One conclusion is inescapable: Women have been catching up with men in the amount of alcohol they drink.

Males still consume more, but the differences between men and women when it comes to drinking are diminishing. Female drinkers are also starting to drink alcohol at an earlier age.

Female alcohol use disorder in the United States more than doubled from 2002 to 2013, according to the National Institute on Alcohol Abuse and Alcoholism. High-risk drinking, defined as more than three drinks in a day or seven in a week for women, rose more than 50 percent in the decade between 2002 and 2013. A 2018 study found a steep rise in the rate of alcohol-related ER visits between 2006 and 2014, and the increase was greater for women than for men. Death from liver cirrhosis rose steadily in women from 2000 to 2013.

It has been a difficult problem to tackle because a woman with a drink problem was not something society looked upon kindly. While men who drank like fish have risen to the top in all walks of life, women have been expected to remain demure, ladylike, and sober. A woman with a drink problem has been unlikely to open up about it, let alone seek help. She would suffer in silence and hope that the problem would go away. Of course, it rarely did.

In recent years, the culture of women and drinking has changed beyond recognition, yet the stigma of alcoholism remains the same. Despite society's acceptance that women are just as entitled to drink as men, problem drinkers still try to hide their condition and hope it will go away.

If that's you, here's some good news:

YOU NO LONGER NEED TO LIVE IN HOPE

You have found a companion to guide you out of the alcohol trap. This book is the key to your escape, a key you can use in complete confidence. When you finish reading it, you will discover that escaping from the tyranny of alcohol is not only possible, it is easy and enjoyable, and you will feel a renewed lust for life.

READING THIS BOOK COULD BE THE BEST DECISION YOU'VE EVER MADE

Alcohol abuse among women is no longer viewed as a problem afflicting the middle classes, if indeed it ever really was. It afflicts young and old, rich and poor, working and nonworking. It is not governed by personality or genes, nor by cultural background, though these factors can influence the way in which the problem drinker suffers. No matter who you are, where you come from, or what you do, no one is immune from the alcohol trap, but once you recognize and accept the trap you are in, escape will be fast and easy. You no longer need to suffer in silence. In fact,

YOU DON'T NEED TO SUFFER AT ALL

BATTLE OF THE SEXES

In the attempt to achieve parity with men, women have sometimes deliberately set out to match, and if possible surpass, the excesses of the other sex. That meant mimicking men's approach to work, to social behavior, to sex, and to drinking. They rightfully trampled triumphantly over sexual inequality. With regard to work, general social behavior, and sex, the result was truly liberating and long overdue. But with regard to alcohol it established a culture whereby it was just as acceptable for a woman to roll out of a bar pie-eyed after an evening's drinking, get into a fight, and fall over, as it is for a man.

From an objective standpoint, you have to question who were the winners in that particular campaign. While women drinkers may have put many a chauvinist in his place, it's come at a price.

> **FACT**
> The death rate among female alcoholics is between 50
> and 100 percent higher than that of male alcoholics.
> *National Institute on Alcohol Abuse and Alcoholism*

Matching the drinking capacity of men may be a badge of honor for a woman drinker, but she is opening herself up to a level of physical abuse way beyond that of her male counterpart. The idea that men have a greater capacity to "hold their drink" than women is not based in chauvinism—though it may be ammunition for chauvinists—it is based in biological fact. One of the key physiological differences between women and men is that the female body contains less water and, therefore, has less capacity to dilute and disperse alcohol. Tragically, the desire to disprove this irrefutable fact has led a multitude of young women into a life of alcohol abuse.

The problem of women drinkers getting younger is widespread. In the United States, where drinking alcohol is illegal under the age of 21, 37 percent of 9th-grade girls (14- and 15-year-olds) admit to drinking in any given month. That's a higher percentage than for boys of the same age. And it's not just one drink. Nearly one in five have consumed more than five drinks in one session—well above the recommended limit for adults.

Maturity may curb the desire to do many stupid things, but it brings new factors that lead many women to drink. As outlined above, studies have revealed that the more educated a woman is and the more senior her position at work, the more likely she is to drink regularly. Factors such as greater exposure to alcohol in childhood, a more active social life, more involvement in traditionally male spheres, and the postponement of childbirth until later in life may all play a part. The bottom line is knowledge; power and affluence are no protection against the alcohol trap. On the contrary, they leave you more vulnerable to the advertising campaigns that blatantly push alcohol to women in the guise of a sophisticated, feminine, empowering lifestyle choice.

In later life too, alcohol is an ever-present threat. Hospitals are admitting as many elderly patients for alcohol-related conditions as for heart attacks, and studies have suggested that women may be more likely than men to develop problems with alcohol in old age. Older women are the biggest users of medication for psychological conditions, such as anxiety and depression, that can react badly when mixed with alcohol. Added to which, the stigma of alcoholism among the older generation is still a major deterrent to seeking help.

MOTHER'S LITTLE HELPER

There are many things in a woman's life these days that can make her feel the need to unwind. More women than ever are going out to work—often being the main breadwinner in a family—and bringing home the stress. We seem to be more "time poor" with each passing year. The increase in opportunity to build a career has not been counter-balanced by an equivalent decrease in maternal obligations. And the competition for jobs, schools, houses, etc. grows increasingly intense.

Relationship problems, depression, and traumas in childhood may also drive you to seek some kind of solace in adulthood, and over the last 30 years or so the form of "stress relief" that has been peddled to women more vigorously than any other is alcohol.

As women have grown more affluent and more independent, the alcohol industry has not been slow to target them as a major growth sector and has advertised its products accordingly. It has also altered the manufacture of its products, concocting new drinks that appeal specifically to the female market and changing the formula of more traditional drinks such as wine to appeal to female tastes.

As a result, more and more women are discovering the misery of becoming a slave to drink. Far from helping to alleviate the pressures of life and making you feel free, it adds a further stress, putting untold strain on relationships, families, purse strings, and health.

THE DAMAGE DONE

You don't need me to tell you about the health risks of excessive alcohol consumption. Cirrhosis of the liver, heart disease, brain disease, and cancer are all strongly linked to alcoholism. Drinking when pregnant can cause brain damage in your child, a condition known as Foetal Alcohol Syndrome. Alcohol suppresses the immune system, leaving you vulnerable to infection and disease; it causes weight gain both through the high calorific value of alcoholic drinks and its tendency to induce hunger; and alcohol consumption frequently leads to smoking, which brings its own set of chronic health risks.

Alcohol impairs judgment, which can be a major risk, particularly to women. It leaves you vulnerable to predatory men, less able to distinguish those with good intentions from those with bad, less able to make sensible choices, and defend yourself physically if the worst comes to the worst.

The rise in the number of women who drink has also been accompanied by a rise in the number of women who drink and drive—and a corresponding increase in the likelihood of causing serious injury or death, either to yourself or someone else, while at the wheel.

> **FACT**
> Drinking and driving has become one of the most common causes of death among women.

WHY YOU WANT TO QUIT

I'm not going to waste your time telling you about the damage that alcohol does to your health: You're already aware of many if not all of the ill effects that alcohol can cause, not only to your health but to your physical and mental wellbeing. This knowledge is not enough to prevent millions of women from continuing to pour alcohol into their system. Nor is it the reason why most drinkers try to quit. Rather it is the everyday miseries that make you wish you could stop: the disrupted sleep, the lack of energy, the inability to deal with stress, the mood swings and depression, the judgment of loved ones and those who care about you.

In short, it's the way alcohol makes you feel. The realization that drinking is not making you happy, it's making you miserable, is what drives most drinkers to attempt to stop. Up to a certain point you'd always felt it had been up to you when and what you drank, but perhaps now an unpleasant realization has begun to creep in:

YOU DON'T CONTROL ALCOHOL, ALCOHOL CONTROLS YOU

Perhaps you've begun to notice some of the classic signs that alcohol has you in its clutches:

- Missing work due to drinking

- Forgetting childcare responsibilities

- Drinking and driving or other behaviors that put you and others at risk

- Embarrassing incidents at work or socially

- Lying about, or concealing, your consumption

- Continuing to drink despite knowing you have a problem

Despite the knowledge that it will do them harm and make them miserable, problem drinkers experience an irresistible craving for alcohol, and once they start drinking they find it very hard to stop. They see alcohol as vile and oppressive but can't understand why they keep falling for it time and time again.

When they do summon the strength to lay off it for a while, they suffer unpleasant withdrawal symptoms, such as the shakes, the sweats, irritability, nausea, and anxiety; and when their willpower gives out and they start drinking again, they find they need bigger and bigger quantities to get any sensation from it at all.

You know full well that you should stop drinking and you feel guilty that you can't, but if someone else tells you that you drink too much, you become defensive and angry. That's because your slavery to alcohol makes you feel helpless, embarrassed, and pathetic. You don't want to be reminded of it by someone else, no matter how well meaning they may be.

A METHOD THAT WORKS

So why can't you just quit? No doubt you've tried to put an end to your drinking in the past and either failed to quit straightaway or been dragged back into the trap after a period of days, weeks, months, or even years. Whatever you've tried before hasn't worked. Why?

Why does it require all your willpower to resist the urge to drink, even though you know it's doing you untold harm, embarrassing you, controlling you, and making you miserable? And why, even if you've managed to abstain for long periods, does that willpower give out and leave you back in the alcohol trap again? No doubt you fall back into the trap by believing that you can "get away" with just having an occasional drink... thinking perhaps that you now have the problem under control. It seems to work for a while, but gradually you get sucked back into the trap even worse than before.

Here's some more good news: You don't need willpower to quit. In fact, as you will learn later in the book, the willpower method actually makes it harder to escape the alcohol trap. Neither do you need to go through a painful withdrawal period. Millions of people succeed in freeing themselves from the alcohol trap without experiencing any pain or unpleasantness whatsoever, and so will you when you finish this book.

It is the belief that quitting has to be hard and painful that prevents most drinkers from escaping from the trap. Imagine you're in a prison with walls ten feet thick, one tiny slit of light high up out of reach, and a heavy iron door that you've been told is almost impossible to open. The first thing you'd do is try to open that door, but, finding it too heavy to budge, you'd soon give up and mope about, convinced that escape is indeed impossible.

That is the state that drinkers find themselves in: trapped in a prison from which they're convinced they cannot escape.

Most drinkers assume they have two choices when it comes to quitting: willpower or Alcoholics Anonymous (AA). In fact, both rely on willpower because they perpetuate the myth that quitting is hard, which in turn reinforces the illusion that alcohol gives you some sort of pleasure or crutch.

This couldn't be further from the truth, which is that

ALCOHOL DOES ABSOLUTELY NOTHING FOR YOU WHATSOEVER

You may already have suspected this but have not yet been convinced. Throughout your life you have been bombarded with misinformation about alcohol and how it eases stress or helps you to enjoy social occasions. You've also been told relentlessly how hard it is to stop drinking. No wonder you find it hard to convince yourself otherwise! It's not just the industries with a vested interested in you drinking that are responsible for this misinformation. It is supported by the very people whose job it is to help you stop: the medical profession and organizations like Alcoholics Anonymous.

AA is an admirable body that has helped a lot of people to turn their lives around after problems with drink, but as any recovering alcoholic who has quit with AA knows, you're in it for the rest of your life. As long as you retain the belief that alcohol does something for you, you will always feel deprived at the thought of having to "give it up" and you will never break free completely.

But what if you were told there was an easy way to open that prison door and given a set of instructions that promised to show you how—you would at least give it a try, wouldn't you? You might be skeptical because you've put all your might into opening that door and you're convinced you don't have the strength. But what's your alternative? To spend the rest of your life trapped in a miserable, dark place?

When I discovered Easyway, a method to cure the world of smoking, easily, painlessly, and permanently, without the need for willpower, I was greeted with skepticism. Yet tens of millions of people have succeeded in quitting smoking as a result of reading Easyway books, attending Easyway centers, watching online webcasts, or using our apps. Millions more turn to Easyway each year for a cure to their addiction, whether it be drugs like nicotine and alcohol, or behavioral addictions like gambling, overeating, and overspending. This global spread has been achieved without ever having to rely on advertising. Easyway has achieved its worldwide success by personal recommendation, for one simple reason:

IT WORKS!

As you begin to read this book it is only natural that all the brainwashing you have been subjected to will make you skeptical. That's fine. There is no harm in questioning what you're told; in fact, I positively encourage it. The reason so many people end up in the alcohol trap is because they don't question what they're told.

Skepticism is perfectly natural at this stage. It will not hamper your attempt to quit provided you don't let it stop you trying. Whatever misgivings you may have at any stage in the book, allow yourself to keep following the method and see where it takes you. There is no great effort involved. And remember the alternative:

to remain trapped in a dark prison for the rest of your life.

Nor do you need to stop drinking yet. You will be given the instruction to take your final drink when you reach the appropriate stage of the book. Until then, make no attempt to change your behavior or do anything that could distract you from taking in everything you read. The one stipulation is that you read the book only when sober. If you've abstained from alcohol for some time, then there is no need to start drinking again; just ignore the references to carrying on drinking and, when it comes to the ritual of the final drink, toward the end of the book, you can just confirm that you have already had yours.

You might be wondering why, if this method is so easy, you can't just skip to the end of the book and uncover the secret. If that were possible, then rest assured we would encourage you to do just that. Nothing could be more convincing than leaping forward in time and seeing how you will feel when you finally free yourself from alcohol, but the method doesn't work like that. If you give in to the temptation to jump ahead, you will fail.

It's like the combination lock on a safe. If we gave you a set of numbers jumbled up on a scrap of paper and you applied them in the wrong order, or you only applied some of them, the lock would remain firmly closed. Easyway is the same. It works by giving you a set of instructions that must be followed in the correct order. Follow all the instructions in order and you cannot fail to get free. That's all it takes. If at any point in the book you forget this and are tempted to skip ahead, come back to this chapter and remind yourself of the first instruction:

FIRST INSTRUCTION:
FOLLOW ALL THE INSTRUCTIONS

SUMMARY

- Women are more likely than men to develop alcohol-related problems
- Alcohol abuse affects all types of women
- Alcohol consumption is a major risk to health and welfare
- Being a slave to alcohol is what drives most attempts to quit
- Quitting doesn't have to be hard—in fact, it's easy
- It's the myths surrounding drinking that make it hard to quit
- Easyway is the only method that makes it easy to quit
- FIRST INSTRUCTION: FOLLOW ALL THE INSTRUCTIONS

Chapter 2

MIND CONTROL

Why do drinkers find it so hard to quit even when they know they're getting no pleasure from it?

We hear many different reasons from women drinkers who come to Easyway centers wanting to quit. Many of them simply say they've grown bored with drinking. It no longer holds any pleasure for them.

There are lots of reasons women turn to alcohol. Statistically, they're twice as likely as men to suffer from depression and anxiety, and are more likely to self-medicate using drink. On the other hand, women often get landed with the short straw in life, and end up being expected to bring up children on their own, or look after elderly parents, or manage the entire household on top of holding down a job. And if they're in a job, they might additionally be trying to fit in with company culture and go out drinking with the men, matching them drink for drink. But the truth is, it usually doesn't take long to see it's making them miserable and they want to gain control of their lives again. Every time they "find themselves drinking" they feel that low, sinking feeling that everyone gets when faced with something mundane.

We all have to do mundane chores from time to time, but if you were told you didn't have to, that there was no point in them, you wouldn't hesitate, you would stop immediately. So why don't women drinkers who have become bored with drinking just stop?

The answer lies in the way the human brain is wired. The rational part of your brain will tell you that drinking is putting you at risk of health problems, wasting your money, and threatening your relationships, and that the logical thing to do is stop, yet the emotional part continues to harbor a desire to drink. The reason the emotional part of your mind doesn't follow the logic of your rational mind is because it's been conditioned to believe a different "truth": that drinking alcohol gives you some sort of pleasure or crutch.

Unfortunately, the emotional mind is often a much stronger influence over your behavior than the rational mind. It governs happiness and the pursuit of happiness is ultimately what governs all our actions. Happiness is the emotion we feel when we satisfy hunger and thirst, or find security and love. These are the base instincts that ensure the survival of our species and happiness is the emotion that drives us to pursue them. So whatever we believe makes us happy is the path we pursue.

Throughout your life you have been told that alcohol gives you some sort of pleasure or crutch. Everywhere you look there are images of smiling, happy people having a drink. Yet in your rational mind you've lost sight of any pleasure in drinking. No matter how hard you try to let the rational side lift you out of the alcohol trap, the conditioning you have experienced keeps dragging you back in. In order to regain control and let your rational mind win the day, you must undo the brainwashing that has created the desire to drink.

ADDICTION

It's easy to undo the brainwashing. First, though, it is essential that you recognize and accept that you have been brainwashed and take a positive attitude to escaping from the trap. It sounds simple, but this is the part that problem drinkers are resistant to and therefore they end up firmly stuck in the trap.

Would you call yourself an alcoholic? The word has a terrible stigma and most of us prefer to think that we haven't yet fallen that far; we just have a little difficulty controlling our drinking. "It's not like I'm addicted or anything."

Let's get one thing straight from the start:

EVERYBODY WHO HAS A DRINK PROBLEM IS ADDICTED

Alcohol is an addictive drug that, like all addictive drugs, hooks you by making you believe it can take away your pain when, in fact, it becomes the reason for your pain. The label of "addict" is not one we assume easily. It conjures up images of junkies, wasting away. But when you understand addiction and how it works, recognizing that you are addicted is the key to your escape.

For me, the moment when everything became clear—and I became free from smoking 100 a day after countless failed attempts to quit—was when I was told that smoking is an addiction. Until then I had seen it as just a habit, a facet of my biological makeup that I somehow lacked the willpower to overcome.

When you see that your problem is addiction, you can dispense with any notion that you are doomed from birth to suffer the problem for life and the route to freedom becomes clear. It's a truly liberating moment.

I called the method Easyway because originally it provided smokers with an easy way to quit smoking. The same method has worked successfully for people with other addictions, including alcohol and other drugs, gambling, overspending, and overeating. The difference between Easyway and all the other methods that claim to help overcome addiction is that the other methods begin with the message that it will *not* be easy. This in itself is another piece of brainwashing that unwittingly keeps addicts in the trap, because the harder you think quitting is going to be, the more fearful you will be of trying and the more you will seek refuge in your addiction. Remember,

THE BELIEF THAT QUITTING WILL BE HARD KEEPS DRINKERS IN THE ALCOHOL TRAP

So let's investigate the reasons why you believe that quitting will be hard.

PROVEN FAILURES

You probably know of other drinkers, or people with other addictions such as smoking or gambling, who have tried to quit but failed. Perhaps you too have tried but found yourself pulled back into the trap by a force that you thought was too strong for you to overcome.

Every failed attempt to quit an addiction is a major setback. Your self-esteem, which is already low because of the helplessness you feel as an addict, takes a further battering. You see your failure as a reflection on yourself and regard yourself as pathetic, weak, and inferior to all those people who appear to sail through life without such problems.

At the same time, you reinforce your belief that your addiction is an impregnable prison from which you will never have the strength to escape.

And it's not only the person who tries and fails to quit who is affected by their failure. Every time you hear of someone who has made an attempt to stop but failed, it reinforces your belief that stopping is incredibly hard. When we look at these people, and even when we look at ourselves, we see people who are, in so many ways, incredibly strong.

Addicts aren't all weak, foolish people. On the contrary, many of the world's most intelligent, strong-minded people have suffered with addiction. Being addicted has nothing to do with lack of willpower. The only reason anyone finds it so hard to escape the alcohol prison is not because it is hard but because they are going about it the wrong way.

LOSING THE WILL

When we say it's essential that you take a positive attitude to escaping from the trap, you may interpret that to mean that you need to draw on all your mental strength. Many people make this assumption, encouraged by the accepted wisdom on addiction from most of the organizations that exist to cure it, but it is a false assumption and one that actually drives addicts further into the trap. After a failed attempt to quit drinking using willpower, you believe that it must be some weakness on your part that prevents you from escaping permanently.

Easyway is the one method for curing addictions that does not tell you to apply willpower. It also happens to be the most effective method ever devised. When you reach the end of this book and experience the elation of finding yourself free, you will know this to be a fact. Right now, however, you may still be finding it hard to believe that you could possibly overcome your addiction without using willpower. That's OK, but remember you have a choice:

1. keep reading and following the instructions and see if we're right

2. continue the way you're going now

Take option one and there is a chance you might escape the misery of alcohol addiction, stop falling deeper and deeper into the trap, losing money, friends, possessions, and self-respect and coming ever closer to the point where you can see absolutely no way of going on. Millions of happy ex-addicts will testify to that chance.

With option 2 there is no chance.

You really have nothing to lose and everything to gain.

Please discount lack of willpower as the reason for any past failures to quit. You failed simply because you were using a method that does not work. If you tried to open a can of soup with a corkscrew, would you blame your lack of willpower when it didn't work? Escaping the alcohol trap is no different. By picking up this book, you have embarked on a method that has been proven to work by millions of people around the world. What's more, it makes it easy. All you have to do is keep reading and follow all the instructions.

THE PERSONALITY MYTH

Just as the belief that quitting will be hard keeps drinkers drinking, so too does the assumption that by "giving up the booze" they will lose a valuable part of their identity. Despite the misery, the slavery, the ill health, the torment, the loss of self-respect, and all the other damaging effects caused by alcohol, some drinkers will continue to see their problem as something that makes them somehow attractive. It just shows how addiction can twist your judgment.

Most drinkers are under the illusion that they become more interesting, wittier, and more fun where they're drinking. But there is another issue at play. Drinking causes us to self-destruct in a way that is deemed attractive... up to a point. Of course, nobody wants to be the dishevelled, incontinent drunk spread-eagled on the sidewalk, but nobody wants to be considered "safe" either.

The word implies boring, unadventurous, predictable. We prefer to be seen as a bit "dangerous"—i.e. exciting, unpredictable, never dull. In popular entertainment, as in life, we tend to feel intimidated by characters who show no vulnerability and we warm to those who are flawed. The tragic character who battles through life against her own demons, be it drink, drugs, gambling, or whatever, usually wins our sympathy and affection over the one who appears to be in complete control and never puts a foot out of place.

We are bombarded with these stereotypes over and over again, and so it's no wonder that our own self-image often can appear more attractive if there are obvious flaws. We worry that if we take the alcohol problem out of our life, we will take on the attributes of the intimidating, invulnerable character and lose what we perceive to be our "charm."

But stop for a second. Isn't it also true that you spend most of your time trying to conceal the fact that you have a drink problem? If your flaws are so charming, why cover them up? It is because we are ashamed of the way drinking affects us. We don't want everybody to know that we have lost control, that we've lost the ability to enjoy life, and that we're stuck in a trap from which we feel incapable of escape.

Get it clear in your mind: There is nothing charming or fanciful about being addicted to alcohol. Cirrhosis of the liver is not charming; nor are stomach ulcers, pancreatitis, gastritis, high blood pressure, strokes, or cancer. There is nothing witty or amusing about anxiety, depression, neurosis, paranoia, and dementia, nor is it endearing to be moody, bad-tempered, unreliable, or untrustworthy.

So if you're being held back from quitting by a belief that you will be less attractive without alcohol in your life, you can let that thought go now. When you quit, you will be amazed how much better you feel: fitter, more confident, more relaxed. All these things will make you more attractive and engaging to those around you, but above all, you will love yourself more.

IN HER OWN WORDS: ANNA

I was still a young girl when my father died from chronic liver damage caused by heavy drinking. It was just after my ninth birthday.

I still have memories of life at home with dad, but at the time I don't think I understood the cause of his condition. What I did understand was the agony and indignity he went through. You would think that would be enough to stop any child from going on to be a drinker, let alone an alcoholic, but when I look back I think I probably saw no other path in life. Once I had tried alcohol and experienced the way it took hold of me, I just saw myself as dad's little girl, destined to go the same way.

Of course, I didn't want to go the same way as dad, and so I did make several attempts to stop drinking, but I never lasted long. The longer I went without a drink, the more I felt I deserved one and soon enough the balance would tip in favor of drinking again. I was under no illusions about the ghastly effect alcohol has on people—I'd seen it with my own eyes—yet I was convinced that I needed alcohol to be the person I wanted to be.

I also convinced myself that nobody else realized how much I was drinking. I thought I had it all under control...

Until one evening after work we went out to celebrate a colleague's birthday and I ended up in the emergency room with a broken jaw, four cracked ribs, and a fractured pelvis. Apparently after drinking too much I'd run straight out in front of a car.

While I was in the hospital, the doctor informed me that he had diagnosed cirrhosis of the liver and that I needed to stop drinking immediately.

I knew what would happen if I didn't and seeing my reflection in the mirror—bruised, bandaged, and pitiful —opened my eyes to the need to find a permanent cure for my drinking. Fortunately for me I found Allen Carr. Until I went to Easyway I was resigned to a life of alcoholism. Now I realize that I have no need for alcohol in my life and I have been free of it for five years. I have literally gotten my life back and it's never been better.

DENIAL

Everyone with a drink problem wishes they could quit. The fact that they can't makes them feel foolish and weak. It's a miserable feeling, so they try to pick themselves up by inventing excuses for why they continue to drink.

"It's just the way I'm made."

"It helps me unwind."

"I just do it to be sociable."

These excuses are just delusions. The implication in each case is that you make a controlled decision to drink, but as everyone who is struggling with a drink problem knows,

YOU DON'T CONTROL ALCOHOL; ALCOHOL CONTROLS YOU

It's a tough thing to have to admit. Having no control over your drinking means society labels you an alcoholic and nobody likes to think of themselves like that. It forces you to face your options: Stay in the trap and continue to suffer the misery, or get out? Getting out seems more frightening than staying in because you've been brainwashed into believing it will be a difficult, painful ordeal and that you will spend the rest of your life feeling deprived. Faced with that prospect, the familiarity of the alcohol trap seems the lesser of two evils.

It's like a tug of war. On one side the fear of what it's doing to you: controlling you, costing you your reputation, your job, your family, your self-respect, your good health, and your energy; on the other is the fear of how you'll cope or even survive without that perceived pleasure or crutch.

FEAR is at both ends of that tug of war. And what is the one thing that causes that fear? ALCOHOL! You've heard of the ostrich that supposedly buries its head in the sand when faced with danger. If you can see the futility of that, you can also see that making excuses just so you don't have to face up to your problem is not going to save you from harm. Once you realize that getting out of the trap doesn't have to be painful or difficult, and you can visualize all the wonderful benefits that come with getting free, the choice becomes easy. You find you're no longer facing two evils—two ends of that tug of war of fear—but one evil and one easy, happy option. Why would anyone choose the former?

THE EASY OPTION

We've talked about the dreadful effects of drinking. The aim is not to scare you into quitting by using shock tactics—that doesn't work and we would not hesitate to use it if it did—but to show you how far the myths about the happy drinker are from the truth. We're more interested in the life that awaits you as a happy nondrinker.

Health

When you're free of alcohol, you will find that you suffer fewer illnesses and recover more quickly when you do fall ill. Your skin, hair, and teeth will look more healthy and your eyes brighter. You will feel less inclined to binge on fast food, so you are likely to lose weight and you will sleep more soundly, giving you more energy and making you less susceptible to stress and anxiety. You will feel aglow with health and happiness. Most women go to incredible lengths to control their weight or lose weight and it's possible that you may have already experienced this during periods when you managed to abstain in the past—when you quit drinking, you lose weight easily. The only thing that may have prevented that in the past is substitution, when perhaps you've tended to eat more in place of drinking alcohol. That just creates misery. In fact, one of the most amazing bonuses of using this method is that because it leaves no feeling of deprivation, there is no compulsion to substitute in any way. I'll explain more about that later.

Control

Regaining control over alcohol also enables you to control other aspects of your life better. You will feel life is less frenetic and you'll be able to make plans that will leave you feeling happy and fulfilled. Life becomes so much more simple when you escape from the alcohol trap. Getting from A to B without having to worry about buses or taxis or getting caught drink-driving; not needing to manipulate friends and family and circumstances and itineraries to ensure you can factor in opportunities or excuses to drink; getting Saturday and Sunday mornings back. It all feels GREAT!

Honesty

Without the requirement for constant excuses and denial that surround life controlled by alcohol you will no longer feel the need to cover your tracks. Dishonesty causes low self-esteem, stress, and anger. When you can look your loved ones in the eye and speak the truth without shame, not to mention look at yourself in the mirror, it will feel like a huge weight being lifted from your shoulders.

Self-respect

Your behavior toward others and the realization that you are no longer a slave to alcohol will make you feel much better about yourself. Every time you think about your achievement in escaping the alcohol trap, you will feel a burst of elation and pride. Rather than being weighed down by a burden of guilt, shame, and embarrassment, you can enjoy freedom, safe in the knowledge that you are in control.

Time

It's hard to find time for everything in life when alcohol is your preoccupation. When you no longer spend your life in search of your next drink or your next phoney excuse to drink, you will find you have so much more time to pursue things that give you genuine pleasure.

Money

Think of the money you will save without alcohol in your life. The average person spends around $90,000 on alcohol in a lifetime. For problem drinkers the figure is a lot higher than that. Think of the genuine fun you could have with that money.

All these wonderful benefits await you when you walk free from the alcohol trap. Escape is easy when you know how. You have already been given the first instruction. The next instruction should help you with everything that follows:

SECOND INSTRUCTION: KEEP AN OPEN MIND

We have talked about the two choices you have: to follow this method and see if it works or to disregard it and stay in the trap. It's an easy choice—all you need to do is keep an open mind.

You might think that's no big deal. Most of us believe we are open-minded. But we are all susceptible to being fooled by preconceptions. Easyway requires you not only to open your mind but to remain aware at all times that there are certain aspects of your mind that may be closed. And then to open them. Take a look at the two tables below, one square, one rectangular.

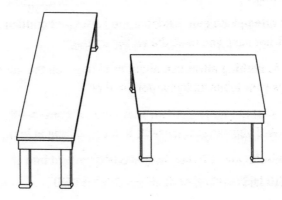

If I were to tell you that the dimensions of each table are exactly the same, you'd be skeptical, wouldn't you? You've already accepted that it's one square table and one rectangular one because that's what I told you it is and it tallies with what you see. But what I told you was a lie; the tables are both identical.

How do you know I'm not lying now? Take a ruler and measure them. Extraordinary, isn't it!

This illusion demonstrates how easily our minds can be tricked into accepting as true something that is false, and how reluctant we are to accept that the opposite might be true. The only way to really know the truth is to check the evidence for yourself. That's what I mean by keeping an open mind: Regardless of what you've believed all your life, always accept that the opposite might be true and don't draw any conclusions until you can see the truth for yourself.

SUMMARY

- You must accept that you are in a trap before you can begin your escape

- Failed attempts to quit reinforce the belief that quitting is hard —that's because you used the wrong methods

- There is nothing attractive about drinking—on the contrary, it destroys your looks and your personality

- Only by facing up to the fear that alcohol causes—the tug of war—will you see that there is, in fact, nothing to fear

- A wonderful new life awaits you when you get free

- SECOND INSTRUCTION: KEEP AN OPEN MIND

Chapter 3

YOUR REASONS FOR DRINKING

Why, despite all we know about the harmful effects of alcohol, do we take up drinking and why do we carry on?

Ask a group of women drinkers why they drink and you will get a range of answers, none of which really explain why we would take a poison that can have a potentially disastrous effect on our health, wealth, relationships, and position in society.

To run a risk of that magnitude surely you must be getting something wonderful in return: an astonishing high, an all-embracing sense of relaxation and joy, a brilliant feeling of happiness.

But that is not the case, is it? On the contrary, drinking makes you feel low, stressed, and frequently miserable! So why do we do it? Let's go back to the start and examine some of the reasons why we take up drinking in the first place. Here are some typical reasons that are given.

"All I wanted to de-stress at the end of the day was a large glass of chilled Chardonnay in my hand."

"I'm a working woman and I wanted to be treated like everyone else. Buying a drink for everybody made me feel like one of the boys, until I found I was going out most days of the week and it began to get me down."

"Alcohol took the rough edges off the world, but the feeling only lasted a short while. Then I realized I was using alcohol in an attempt to mask my real feelings. Alcohol doesn't solve anything."

We all know that, even in so-called normal drinkers, alcohol debilitates all the bodily functions, in particular the senses and coordination. Rather than putting us off, this feature of alcohol is actually made out to be one of the attractions, especially among young people who are relatively new to drinking.

"I got totally battered last night."

"I want to get sloshed."

"Let's get hammered."

These common expressions speak of serious physical impairments. Why would we want to inflict such damage on ourselves? As children, with relatively little knowledge, we content ourselves with innocent games. As adults, with more knowledge, we deliberately put ourselves in the way of harmful pursuits. It's a paradox that is caused by a psychological condition that affects everyone to a certain extent, an emptiness that opens up during our development, starting from birth. We call it "the void" and it affects all of us to different degrees.

The shock of birth leaves us desperately seeking security. We reach for our mothers and they protect us. Our neediness and vulnerability continue through childhood, when we're cocooned from the harsh realities of life in a fantasy world of make-believe. But before long we discover that Santa Claus and fairies do not exist. Worse still, we discover that life isn't forever. Consciousness of our own mortality is frightening. At the same time we're forced from the safety of home to school and to a new set of fears and insecurities. As we enter our teens, we look more critically at our parents and it begins to dawn on us that they are not the unshakeable pillars of strength that we had always thought them to be. They have weaknesses, frailties, and fears, just as we do. We call it growing up and toughening up, but while we may develop a tough outer shell, the disillusionment leaves a void in our lives. We attempt to fill that void with other role models: pop stars, models, actresses, TV celebrities, sportswomen. Enchanted by their seemingly glamorous, exciting, fulfilling lifestyles, we revere these people, and regard them as the perfect template for our own lives. We try to bask in their reflected glory. Instead of becoming strong, complete, secure, and unique individuals in our own right, we become followers, impressionable fans, leaving ourselves wide open to suggestion. Whatever they do, we want to copy them. We might not be able to drive an expensive car, go on lavish vacations, or live in big houses, but we can afford a drink and a smoke. Watch the way smokers hold a cigarette and drinkers hold a glass. They're all mimicking somebody. In many ways, it's the closest we can get to the lifestyle we dream of.

CELEBRITY ROLE MODELS

Celebrities are mostly unaware of the power they hold. The label "role model" is one that many would rather disassociate themselves from, such is the burden of responsibility. They just want to live their lives without having to worry about the effect they have on people they don't know. Understandable perhaps—after all, all celebrities begin as "normal people." But the plain truth is that their actions can and do affect millions. Drinking is as much a part of the high society lifestyle as it ever was, and among women it has increased dramatically. In the early days of modern showbiz, it was deemed unladylike for a woman to be seen drunk; today, the sight of a female celebrity falling out of a nightclub and into a car is a weekly occurrence. Does this dissuade impressionable young girls from drinking? On the contrary, it reinforces the myth that drinking is "the thing to do."

THE SOCIAL DRUG

Another major influence is our circle of friends. Regardless of what we might think privately about alcohol, when all our friends are drinking we come under pressure to join in. Alcohol, after all, is perceived as the sociable drug, the drug we take in groups so we can all get drunk together. Anyone who stands apart from that accepted norm is seen as a party pooper, or at least they perceive themselves to be.

Among adults, drinking, unlike any other form of drug taking, is considered normal behavior and those who don't drink are regarded as the exception. So not only do we have the influence of our role models encouraging us to drink, we also have the pressure of our peer group. It's in our nature to want to fit in, and so we drink and we drink and we push all the facts we know about the harmful effects of alcohol to the back of our minds.

In fact, in a twisted way our knowledge of the harm that alcohol causes actually becomes a reason to drink. As young adults we all want to prove that we can handle danger because we perceive that as something adults do. It's no longer just young men who show off over the amount they can drink. Young women do it too and now they get plenty of encouragement from their friends.

But there is a further, more subtle way in which the known harm caused by drinking can actually attract us to it: the promise of an unknown pleasure. During our teenage years we discover that lots of things we've been warned against are actually pleasurable. This sows a seed in our minds: We suspect that this might be the case with everything we've been warned against. Then we see people we admire enjoying those very things and our suspicions are confirmed.

Subconsciously we ask ourselves the same question that we asked at the beginning of this chapter: "OK, so booze can leave you destitute, derelict, even dead, but to run a risk of that magnitude surely you must be getting something wonderful in return?" And so we go in pursuit of the unknown pleasure.

The simple truth, which we are never told, is that all those influences—the celebrities, the friends, our parents—are drinking because they too have been brainwashed and now they can't stop. They never found the unknown pleasure and they never will simply because

THERE IS NO PLEASURE

WHY WE CONTINUE TO DRINK

We first start drinking because we believe there must be something pleasurable in doing so. We're not sure what that pleasure is, but we don't want to miss out. That first drink tastes foul. If you took that drink without any of the brainwashing that came before it, you would spit it out and never go near it again. But because you believe in the unknown pleasure you persevere. Against all your natural responses, you continue to drink this foul poison until you no longer find the taste repulsive.

Aware of the obstacle that this process places in the way of a young drinker's, particularly of the female variety, journey to "full drinker" status, the alcohol industry has conspired to create a whole new generation of alcoholic drinks designed to smooth the way. Initially in the form of alcopops, alcoholic lemonade, ginger beer, and sodas, and more recently in the form of sickly sweet fruit ciders or wine coolers or fluorescent-colored "shots," the products have provided a much less harsh "entry level" drink for youngsters who only have to get over the ghastly sweetness rather than the far less palatable hard liquors and beers that their 1960s, 1970s, and 1990s counterparts had to endure. Even so, those youngsters still look like they're taking medicine rather than enjoying a beverage when you watch them taking their first drinks.

It's an extraordinary process to go through, yet 90 percent of adults go through it, and all for the promise of the nonexistent unknown pleasure. We don't expect that pleasure to come easily or immediately. We're told that alcohol is an acquired taste and we grow up perceiving adults to be resilient and strong-willed. They don't give up easily. If they think something's worth fighting for, they'll fight for it. If we are to be perceived as adults, we need to follow suit.

"Acquiring a taste" for alcohol may be a revolting ordeal, but we're not about to give in at the first hurdle. We shall overcome! We are convinced that there is some amazing pleasure to be had from drinking because we see it throughout society. If we didn't experience it the first time, well, we'll just have to try harder, won't we?

YOU CONTINUE TO DRINK BECAUSE YOU'RE CHASING AN IMPOSSIBLE GOAL

That goal is the achievement of the unknown pleasure. Until you experience that pleasure, you feel unfulfilled. Over time, as you feel less repulsed by the taste, drinking does seem to become more pleasurable, and so you conclude that the more you go on drinking, the closer you will get to your goal. In truth, the opposite is true. The more you drink, the further you get from ever feeling a sense of fulfillment. That is the nature of drug addiction. It keeps you on the hook by never allowing you to feel completely satisfied.

ONLY BY QUITTING ALCOHOL CAN YOU FEEL FULFILLED

The only reason alcohol tastes less repulsive with practice is because you build up a tolerance to the poison. It is not an "acquired taste," it is an acquired loss of taste. The human body has the incredible capacity to build its own resistance to poisons by shutting down the faculties that try to fight them. Your reaction to your first drink was your body trying to expel poison; with continued use, these defenses are knocked out and the alcohol slips by unchecked. It's like letting gatecrashers into your party. You might avoid an ugly scene at the door, but you leave yourself wide open to having your house wrecked.

THE ILLUSION OF PLEASURE

Building a tolerance against alcohol doesn't make drinking a pleasure; it just makes it less of a "displeasure." We think we are acquiring a taste for it and this reinforces our belief that drinking is a pleasure. At the same time we develop a craving for alcohol. Horrible though it is, that first drink is all it takes to trigger the downward spiral that leads to chronic alcoholism. I'll explain later why some people become alcoholics and others don't, but at this stage all that matters is that you accept that it has nothing to do with the drinker and everything to do with the drink.

Alcohol is a highly addictive drug. As it passes out of your system it leaves a feeling of unease and emptiness, like a niggling itch, not dissimilar to hunger. It's barely perceptible. Just as you interpret hunger as the need for food, you interpret the withdrawal from alcohol as "I need a drink." The only way to seemingly get rid of it is to have one and thus the cycle of addiction begins.

When you have your next drink, the feeling of unease and emptiness is partially relieved, giving the impression of a little boost. We call this the illusion of pleasure. It's just the ending of a dissatisfied condition created by the first drink. But that's not real pleasure—it's like wearing tight shoes just for the relief of taking them off. You mistake this little boost for pleasure and, because you're not aware that alcohol was the cause of your discomfort, it becomes ingrained in your mind that alcohol gives you pleasure.

When drinkers say they drink for the high it gives them, what they're talking about is nothing more than the relief of taking off tight shoes. Would you wear tight shoes all day just for the "pleasure" of taking them off? Don't get me wrong—no doubt you might wear all kinds of shoes which cause you all kinds of pain—but remember that has nothing to do with the feeling of taking them off and everything to do with the way they look. You simply wouldn't wear a pair of tight shoes JUST for the relief of taking them off. What drinkers are enjoying, in fact, is coming close to the feeling of normality that a nondrinker feels all the time. Without alcohol you don't suffer the uncomfortable, insecure feeling in the first place.

THE FULFILLMENT ALL DRINKERS SEEK IS FEELING HOW A NONDRINKER FEELS ALL THE TIME

THE ONLY WAY YOU CAN DO THAT IS NOT TO DRINK

As long as you keep drinking, you will never feel fulfilled. Addiction is like a fruit machine that has been "fixed" so that it is guaranteed never to pay out what you put into it. All drinkers want to get back to "break-even"—the way they felt before they ever started drinking—but they are deluded into thinking the only way to do that is to drink more. If you can see the folly in a gambler pumping coins into that fraudulent fruit machine, you can see that drinking to feel like a nondrinker makes just as little sense.

THE PURSUIT OF HAPPINESS

We are brainwashed into believing that alcohol gives us some sort of pleasure or crutch, but when you examine the feelings that drive us to drink they all have a very negative theme:

- Boredom—"It's something to do and it keeps my mind occupied."

- Sadness—"It helps me forget that I'm alone."

• Stress—"It helps me to chill out and forget about my worries."

• Routine—"It's just what I do when the kids have gone to bed."

• Reward—"It's my treat after a long, hard day."

Happiness doesn't come into it. True, we mark happy occasions with a celebratory drink, but that is nothing more than a custom. We don't feel a need or desire for that drink. In fact, it is when we are happiest that our desire for a drink is least. Next time you're at a wedding, take note of all the unfinished glasses of champagne left on the tables when the dancing begins.

If drinking is a pleasure, why wait until you're bored or sad or stressed to do it? A yoga class is a pleasure for many people—they don't wait until they're bored, sad, or stressed before they go and do yoga. They might do it at the same time on the same day every week, but it's not the routine that compels them to go. "It's Wednesday evening. I have to go to yoga. I have no choice." On the contrary, they can't wait for Wednesday evening to come around and would happily break their routine to do it sooner if they could.

The illusion of pleasure is intertwined with the illusion of reward. If you think something gives you pleasure, you will use it to reward yourself. You might make time for an extra yoga class or you might have a drink. One is a genuine pleasure and will leave you feeling good; the other is a false pleasure and will leave you feeling low. The confusing thing is that drinkers know this. They know how drinking makes them feel and they know the harm it can cause, yet they continue to kid themselves that it gives them pleasure or a crutch. This confusion makes you feel helpless and stupid. That's because you haven't been given the true picture.

Remember the tables in the last chapter: When you were told they were the same and you double-checked, you were able to convince yourself easily, but until the truth was pointed out to you, you were convinced they were different.

You've been told all your life that alcohol gives you some sort of pleasure or support and you've convinced yourself that this is why you continue to drink. Nobody has told you that you are, in fact, caught in an ingenious trap and that is the only reason you continue to drink.

Until now.

Let's take a closer look at the trap.

```
┌------------------  SUMMARY  ------------------┐
|                                               |
| • Role models help to convince us that alcohol will fulfill our
|   desire for pleasure or a crutch             |
|                                               |
| • Only a nondrinker can be sure of not having an alcohol problem
|                                               |
| • The only way to feel fulfilled like a nondrinker is not to drink
|                                               |
| • The illusion of pleasure is relief and nothing more
|                                               |
| • Genuine pleasures need no excuses           |
|                                               |
| • The only reason you continue to drink is that you are caught in
|   a trap                                      |
|                                               |
└-----------------------------------------------┘
```

Chapter 4

A SUBTLE TRAP

The alcohol trap awaits everyone who starts drinking and it affects them all in the same way. You need to understand how it works in order to escape.

The illusion of pleasure is merely partial relief from the craving for alcohol. The craving is caused by the alcohol from the last drink leaving your system. Therefore, it should follow that if you can go long enough for all the alcohol to pass out of your body, the craving should stop and your addiction will be cured.

As every drinker knows, this is not the case. It takes no more than one hour on average for the liver to metabolize one unit of alcohol and about a week to ten days for the body to rid itself of all the toxins. Plenty of drinkers have managed to go a lot longer than ten days without a drink, but they've still found themselves dogged by the craving. In fact, the craving has gotten worse. They need all their willpower to resist it, but eventually it becomes too much for them and they start drinking again.

Blood Alcohol Content (BAC)

Blood Alcohol Content is the weight of ethanol (alcohol), measured in grams, in 100 milliliters of blood. It burns off at 0.015 BAC an hour or roughly one unit of alcohol per hour. The rate remains the same for everybody, male or female, large or small. What varies, however, is the rate at which your BAC increases. It can take a large male five drinks or more in an hour to reach a BAC of 0.08 (at which point many countries consider you legally intoxicated), whereas a small female might reach the same level with far less.

Women's bodies don't process alcohol as efficiently as men's. Several biological factors make women more vulnerable. First, women tend to weigh less than men, and—pound for pound—a woman's body has less water and more fatty tissue than a man's. Because fat retains alcohol while water dilutes it, a woman's organs sustain greater exposure. In addition, women have lower levels of the enzymes that break alcohol down in the stomach and liver.

When drinking similar amounts, women will retain more alcohol in their blood and take longer to expel it from their bodies than men and therefore the effects are likely to be longer-lasting and more harmful.

(Thanks to *Harvard Health*)

IN HER OWN WORDS: JAN

I managed to stop drinking in April and I was doing really well. Plenty of occasions came and went when I could have had a drink, but I managed to resist and I was feeling really pleased with myself.

Then Christmas came. At the start of December I could feel myself getting into Christmas mode and something inside me started craving a drink. Whether it was the stress of all the preparation or just the time of year being traditionally a time when I would have drunk a lot, I don't know, but I decided to allow myself a glass of wine.

The next thing I knew I'd drained the whole bottle and was back to square one. I couldn't believe I'd caved in so easily, but if I'm honest, during the seven months I'd been dry, I hadn't gone a single day without wanting a drink. When I finally opened that bottle of wine, it was like welcoming an old lover back into my house—a lover I knew would smash the place up and run off with my money.

Purging your body of alcohol would be the simple cure if the problem was purely physical, but there are two aspects to addiction: a physical aspect (the mild physical withdrawal) and a mental aspect, and the mental aspect is far more powerful. The physical aspect is like a little monster in your body that cries feebly when it's running out of alcohol. The feeling is not painful—you feel it after every session. It is nothing worse than a small itch, a feeling of not being quite right within yourself, but it is enough to arouse the Big Monster in your mind, which interprets those feeble cries as "I need a drink." Until you satisfy the Big Monster, you will suffer a feeling of deprivation. It is the Big Monster that makes you irritable when you can't drink. It's the Big Monster that makes you feel worse and worse, the longer you go without a drink, and it is the Big Monster that makes you feel relief when you get a drink in your hand.

The craving is 1 percent physical and 99 percent mental. It takes six minutes for alcohol to take effect on your nervous system, yet the relief you feel when you finally get a drink is instantaneous. The Big Monster isn't pacified when it feels the alcohol coming through your bloodstream; it's pacified as soon as it knows it's coming. Think about it. Often the cravings disappear the moment you decide to have another drink, or the moment you walk into the bar, or the instant you begin to open the bottle of wine—the alcohol hasn't even touched your lips yet the discomfort has disappeared! Those unpleasant panic feelings, the anxiety, the irritability have nothing to do with alcohol withdrawal and everything to do with what is going on in your mind. They are real physical feelings, but it's important to understand that they have no physical cause. They are generated by a thought process. Don't be intimidated by this fact—it's fabulous news! It simply means that once we've gotten rid of that Big Monster, the rest is plain sailing.

When you use willpower to stop drinking, the Big Monster lives on long after all the alcohol has left your system because it doesn't rely on alcohol for survival—it relies on fear, illusions, and myths. It was created by all the brainwashing that led you to believe that alcohol gives you some sort of pleasure or crutch. It was further nurtured by you mistakenly believing that each drink got rid of the slight physical withdrawal (mistaking that feeling for pleasure or relief) rather than realizing that the discomfort was created by your first drinks (it simply wasn't there before you started drinking and nondrinkers never experience it) and becoming blind to the fact that each subsequent drink perpetuated the discomfort. As long as you go on believing that, the Big Monster will continue to hold you in its clutches. Understand how it works and that Big Monster is slain.

The Big Monster plays an ingenious trick. It convinces you, through the illusion of pleasure, that the only thing that can relieve your craving is the thing that caused it in the first place. Thus it guarantees that you remain trapped in a cycle of addiction from which there is no escape as long as the Big Monster remains alive. In order to kill the Big Monster, you just need to unravel the brainwashing. That's what Easyway does. Some people describe Easyway as brainwashing—in fact it's the opposite—it's counter-brainwashing.

Imagine brainwashing being like a rubber band wound around two pencils and the pencils being twisted around in opposite directions tighter and tighter and tighter over time. What Easyway does, by explaining the myths and illusions that surround addiction, is gradually, gently, slowly, to unwind the rubber bands, so that the pencils can be separated again. One pencil is called FACT; the other is called FICTION; and separating them is called COUNTER-BRAINWASHING. By merely having an open frame of mind you are simply stopping the twisting of the rubber band in the direction that tightens the bond, and gently allowing the bands to loosen. Let it happen. It takes no effort.

GAMBLING ADDICTS

The mental aspect of addiction becomes very clear when you look at an addiction like gambling, one of the most chronic addictions gripping the world in the 21st century. Gambling does not involve ingesting a substance, like alcohol, nicotine, or heroin, yet problem gamblers show all the same symptoms as drinkers, smokers, and heroin addicts. It is the illusion of pleasure that hooks them all.

THE PITCHER PLANT

The alcohol trap is so subtle in its cunning that drinkers fall for it without even realizing. An apt comparison is the pitcher plant, that pitcher-shaped marvel of nature that feeds on flies that wander unwittingly into its digestive chamber. The fly lands on the rim of the plant and begins to feed. The nectar tastes good—it seems like the best thing in the world—but it's a bait, luring the fly closer and closer to death. The more the fly feeds, the further down the pitcher it wanders, the sides getting steeper and steeper, until it loses its grip and falls in to the digestive fluid at the bottom.

All addictions work in a similar way to the pitcher plant, once you're in the trap. Whereas the fly is drawn to the nectar

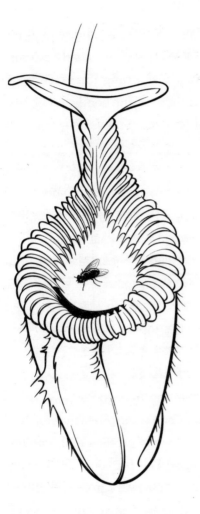

by instinct, we are drawn to alcohol by brainwashing. And while the fly's love of nectar is natural and immediate, we have to persevere for a while until the taste of alcohol no longer makes us gag. But by this stage we are in the trap.

WE'RE ALREADY LOSING CONTROL

The pride we feel in being grown-up enough to take our drink draws us to alcohol as the nectar draws the fly. We relish every opportunity to drink but still feel in control of when and how much we drink. We're confident that there will be no problems.

The fly is confident too, right up to the point where it realizes that it's trapped. At that point it's already too late: There is no escape. Why doesn't it fly away before it gets trapped? Why does it stay and continue to drink? Because it has no idea what lies ahead.

Some people can't bear to watch a fly in a pitcher plant.

They want to intervene, to flick the fly away and save it from its inevitable end. You might feel the same if you saw a heroin addict. You would want to intervene and save her from the terrible decline that you can see coming but she can't.

A NONDRINKER WOULD FEEL
THE SAME WAY ABOUT YOU

THE INEVITABLE DECLINE

Addiction drives us to seek relief from the craving in the very thing that caused the craving in the first place. But the relief is not complete. Not all of the craving is satisfied. This comes back to the body's ability to build a defensive tolerance to poison. As that tolerance builds up, you need to take bigger and bigger doses of the poison to have the same effect. Because of this we never get back to the feeling of normality that a nondrinker feels all the time. How can we when each and every drink only partially relieves the withdrawal as our physical and mental health is continuously declining? It still feels like you get a boost when you drink, but it's a con trick, like wearing tight shoes just for the relief of taking them off.

THE ONLY WAY TO TRULY FEEL LIKE A NONDRINKER
IS TO BECOME ONE

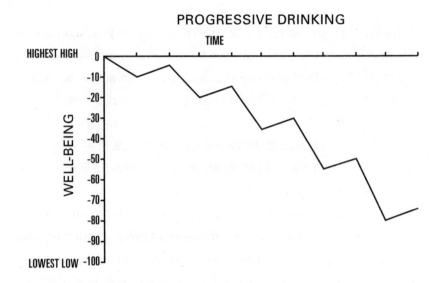

This graph illustrates the inevitable decline of the alcohol addict. The nondrinker's "normal" is at 0. A drinker in the early stages is at -5 because of a combination of the withdrawal and the decline in mental and physical health. The next drink boosts you back up to -1. You do feel better than a moment before, but you don't get back to 0. And so the trap is set. The next withdrawal takes you down 5 points again to -6 and the next drink, because your tolerance is increasing and you never fully relieve the withdrawal, boosts you up only to -3. With each drink your level of normal is slipping, just as the fly slips down the pitcher plant. Yet you still experience that boost. It's no wonder you think you get something from alcohol. It's an ingenious, subtle trap.

The next thing that happens is that your fall starts to accelerate. In addition to the physical low comes a mental low brought about by the Big Monster that now convinces you that you do actually feel better every time you drink. When you try to ignore it, it creates havoc, demanding its next fix. The longer you resist, the more it stamps its feet and the greater the boost seems when you finally cave in. This in turn makes the Big Monster bigger and more powerful. In order to overcome your tolerance and satisfy the Big Monster, you need to increase the dose. The bigger the dose, the deeper the low, so now the falls are increasing and the boosts are getting smaller.

And so you go on, falling by ever-increasing amounts. While each little boost continues to mislead you into believing that drinking is giving you some sort of pleasure or crutch, the reality is that you're becoming increasingly miserable. You can see the effect that drinking is having on you and you feel confused and weak at your inability to curb it. This creates a triple low: the physical and mental lows, plus the misery of knowing you are hooked on booze. No matter how low the drug drags you down, you remain grateful for the "boost" it gives you as it drags you deeper and deeper into the trap. Deep down inside, you know that you've become a slave to alcohol.

THE ADDICTION HAS TAKEN HOLD

CONTROL

The fly doesn't escape the pitcher plant because it can't see the danger until it's too late. Right up until that point it believes it's in control. When it tries to fly free, it finds it can't; it's stuck, and it's just a matter of time before it slips to its death.

The fact is the fly was never in control. It was being controlled by the plant from the moment it first caught the aroma of the nectar. The same is true of all drinkers.

YOU DON'T CONTROL ALCOHOL; ALCOHOL CONTROLS YOU

You are controlled from the moment you're drawn to that first drink, but, like the fly, you only realize you're in the trap when you're well and truly hooked. It's an unpleasant realization that creates further anxiety and so you reach for the one thing that you think can ease your stress: booze.

Until you can see and understand the nature of the trap you're in, the misery of knowing you're controlled by alcohol will not make you stop; it will make you drink more. This is how addiction works.

THE ADDICT SEEKS RELIEF IN THE VERY THING THAT'S CAUSING THE MISERY

WHAT'S STOPPING YOU FROM FLYING FREE

To a nondrinker the solution looks simple: Stop drinking and just fly free. But when you're actually in the trap, nothing looks simple. The Big Monster blinds you to reality with two myths:

1. The myth that drinking gives you pleasure and/or a crutch.

2. The myth that escape will be hard and painful.

The second instruction was to keep an open mind. Since you were young you have been led to believe that alcohol gives you some sort of pleasure or crutch; that it lubricates social occasions, makes you more relaxed and eloquent; that it eases stress and obliterates sadness. Now consider this:

ALCOHOL DOES ABSOLUTELY NOTHING FOR YOU WHATSOEVER

Remember to keep an open mind. Like most people, you no doubt have good memories of happy occasions when you've drunk heavily: parties, celebrations, weekends away with friends. You may feel that these occasions wouldn't have been the same without alcohol. But look again—where did the real pleasure come from on those occasions? Was it the drinking that made your day? Or was it the company of friends, the chats you had, the sheer pleasure of being with people you like?

Take away the drinking and the situation would still have been enjoyable. Take away the company and the drinking would have been no fun.

How can a poison that causes irritability, impatience, loss of memory, nausea, and headache make life more fun? Equally, how can a poison that causes stress, anxiety, self-pity, and lack of judgment be a crutch to help you cope with the pressures of life?

We believe these myths because they are drummed into us from a young age and reinforced by the illusion of pleasure—that combination of the Little Monster and the Big Monster. Question everything you've been told and led to believe throughout your life and recognize the illusion of pleasure for what it is—nothing more than partial relief, like the "pleasure" of wearing tight shoes just for the relief of taking them off—and the myth that alcohol gives you pleasure or a crutch is easy to dispel.

The myth that quitting will be hard and painful is also created by brainwashing and reinforced by failed attempts to quit—both yours and those of other people you know. Those failed attempts were due to using the wrong methods. When you quit with Easyway there is no need for willpower and there is no painful withdrawal period. It's easy!

Wherever you may be on the inevitable decline into the alcohol trap, there is good news for you. You may feel like the fly, doomed to slide into oblivion, but there is one crucial difference between the fly in the pitcher plant and your fate in the alcohol trap:

IT'S NOT TOO LATE FOR YOU TO ESCAPE FROM THE ALCOHOL TRAP

All those increasing lows on the graph are recoverable when you quit drinking. Millions of people, who have found themselves in the same trap and been convinced that they will never be able to escape, have gotten free and so will you. It has nothing to do with your character, or personality, or willpower.

You are not standing on a slippery slope; there is no physical force compelling you to drink more. The trap is entirely in your mind. One of the ingenious aspects of addiction is that it makes you your own jailer, but that, fortunately for you, is also its fatal flaw. You have the power to escape any time you choose. All you have to do is kill the Big Monster by unraveling the brainwashing and removing the desire for alcohol. Doing that is simple and easy and just requires you to carry on reading and following all the instructions.

SUMMARY

- **Addicts seek relief in the very thing that's causing the problem**
- **With each "boost" you fall a little further**
- **The illusion that alcohol provides pleasure or a crutch and the myth that it is hard to escape keep you trapped**
- **It's never too late to fly free and recapture the joy of being a nondrinker**

Chapter 5

FIRST STEPS TO FREEDOM

The brainwashing creates a perception of alcohol that makes escape seem impossible. Unravel the brainwashing and the way out becomes clear.

For a drinker who has tried and failed to quit, the alcohol trap feels like a prison from which you can never escape. This can have a terrible effect on your desire to stop drinking. If you believe you stand no chance of stopping, what's the point in trying? We see the same mindset in all kinds of addicts: drinkers, smokers, gamblers —resignation to a life of misery. Compared to the frustration and humiliation of repeated failed attempts to quit, it often appears the least painful option.

The mistake these addicts all make is trying to find excuses or reasons why they drink. They don't realize that the drug has them in a trap and that alone means they always draw the wrong conclusions. It reinforces the Big Monster. The first step to freedom from the prison is recognizing that drinking is not just a habit that you can't seem to kick because you like it; it's addiction. Then you can understand the true nature of the trap.

Recognizing that you are an addict changes your whole way of looking at the problem. For the first time you can see that it's not a weakness in your character that has kept you hooked; nor is it some magical quality in the drink. When you see these two crucial facts, the feeling of powerlessness and resignation goes and you realize that escape is within your grasp.

Women and Addiction

- Women addicts often use addictive substances such as alcohol or cocaine in an attempt to self-medicate when they are feeling low, while generally speaking men tend to use them when they feel good in an attempt to feel even better.
- Women are less likely to develop drug- and drink-related problems, but when they do develop such problems, they tend to develop them faster.
- When women do develop substance abuse problems, they report worse related consequences.

By every quantitative measure, women are drinking more.

Women are being charged more often with drunk driving, they're more frequently measured with high concentrations of alcohol in their bloodstreams at the scene of car accidents, and they're more often treated in hospital emergency rooms for intoxication.

Men's drinking, arrests for drunk driving, and alcohol purchases remain stagnant or are even decreasing.

In the past ten years record numbers of women have sought treatment for alcohol abuse.

WHAT IS ADDICTION?

Every type of addiction works in the same way. The effect of the drug distorts your natural coping mechanisms, so you turn more and more to the drug for the perceived pleasure or crutch and become less and less able to live without it. Of course, not all addictions involve a drug like alcohol or nicotine. They don't need to: addiction is 99 percent mental. For gamblers, for example, the act of betting money has the same effect on certain parts of the brain as the intrusion of alcohol or nicotine. It replaces genuine pleasure with a false pleasure, which you can only attain by continuing to gamble, drink, smoke, or whatever.

The pursuit of that false pleasure sends you deeper and deeper into the trap, since each "fix" needs to be stronger than the one before. The further in you go, the more you lose sight of genuine pleasures. You find that all you're living for is the next fix. If you can't have it, you feel deprived. The sense of deprivation is a miserable feeling and the longer it goes on, the worse it gets.

Feeling powerless to stop drinking despite the harm you know it's causing you is a sure sign of addiction. As with all addictions, it's the illusion that the drug provides a genuine pleasure or crutch that keeps you trapped. Drinkers suffer from the illusion that alcohol helps them relax, gives them courage, makes them more eloquent and fun to be with. In fact, it does the complete opposite.

ALCOHOL DOES ABSOLUTELY NOTHING FOR YOU WHATSOEVER!

When you open your mind to this simple truth, it naturally follows that stopping drinking involves no sacrifice or deprivation. Quitting becomes easy, immediate, and permanent.

HOW EASYWAY WORKS

When people first hear about Easyway, they want to know what is the secret of this magical cure. We have to tell them:

1. It is not a secret

2. There is no magic

Easyway is a method that works by using plain logic to unravel the brainwashing that leads us into the alcohol trap and replaces it with a clear, rational understanding of the problem, which in turn removes the desire to drink. The key to the method is the set of instructions that you are given throughout the book and it must be used like the combination lock of a safe: Each instruction must be understood and applied in order for the door to eventually spring open.

Your first instruction was to follow all the instructions. Your second was to keep an open mind. In getting this far we can assume that you have followed those two instructions and are ready for your third. Please be patient. As explained in Chapter One, the key to your escape does not lie in the final chapter or the first chapter, or any chapter alone; the whole book is the key.

THE DIFFERENCE BETWEEN DRINKERS AND NONDRINKERS

Drinkers and smokers are notorious for "giving up" and starting again. For some people it becomes a running joke. Of course, quitting temporarily isn't quitting at all. You are still hooked, you are still a slave, and you are still unhappy. In fact, during those temporary suspensions in drinking you are less happy than when you're drinking because you still crave a drink, but you can't have one. As I'll explain in more detail later in the book, stopping and starting actually reinforces your desire to drink.

For those drinkers who make a joke of stopping and starting, drinking has become a fact of life, something they don't question. Such is the brainwashing, they believe that their slavery to alcohol is perfectly normal. In fact, they kid themselves that it's an endearing part of their character. Too bad it makes them feel miserable.

From an early age we are fed a false view of reality, just as we misled you about the tables in Chapter Two. We are led to believe that drinking gives some sort of pleasure or crutch. By now your mind should be open to the possibility that the opposite is true. You may not be convinced of it yet, but you should at least be prepared to be convinced. If you're not, you haven't followed the second instruction. Go back and look at the table illusion again and accept that the truth isn't always what you perceive it to be. It's easy to be misled by false information.

Now bear in mind that 10 percent of adults have lived their lives without ever falling for the alcohol trap. They too have been subjected to a massive amount of brainwashing, but for some reason they haven't fallen for it. This brings us to the difference between drinkers and nondrinkers.

The obvious difference is that one drinks and the other doesn't, but that doesn't complete the picture for us. We need to know why the brainwashing works on some people and not on others.

Stand a drinker and a nondrinker side by side and put a drink in their hands. The drinker will find it very hard not to take a sip, whereas the nondrinker will put the drink aside without any problem at all. What has compelled them to act as they do? No one forces the drinker to drink, but it takes all her willpower not to. The force that compels her to drink is desire and that is the crucial difference between drinkers and nondrinkers:

NONDRINKERS NEVER HAVE THE DESIRE TO DRINK

Easyway helps you to become a nondrinker for life by removing your desire to drink.

How have that 10 percent who live their lives without ever falling for the alcohol trap or developing the desire to drink avoided it? They've been subjected to the same brainwashing as you, so somewhere in their minds they will believe that there is some benefit to be enjoyed from drinking. They too may have been tempted, but, like you, they will also be aware of the harm that alcohol can cause. Thinking rationally, they see no sense in inflicting that on themselves. Even if they do try it, they find the taste disgusting and are not prepared to work at "acquiring the taste."

From that you might deduce that you became hooked because you lacked the power of reason to outweigh temptation. In fact, there are countless reasons why you might have made that decision to pursue the unknown pleasure of drink. Remember, all adults have a 90 percent chance of doing the same. The important thing is that you now know the unknown pleasure is an illusion and that knowledge gives you a distinct advantage.

When you escape the alcohol trap with Easyway, you are actually less vulnerable to falling for it in future than someone who has never been a drinker. For them the belief that drinking gives some sort of pleasure or crutch is still there in their mind; they just haven't chosen to find out because the arguments against drinking outweigh the temptation as far as they can judge. But their judgment could change. A trauma of some kind could see them turning to drink at any point in their life, believing it will give them the pleasure or support they need. For the nondrinker who has quit with Easyway, that belief no longer exists.

EASYWAY DOES NOT REQUIRE THE POWER OF REASON TO OUTWEIGH TEMPTATION; IT REMOVES TEMPTATION ALTOGETHER

Take away the desire to drink and you remove the sense of sacrifice and deprivation that leads to temptation. Drinkers only think removing the desire to drink will be hard because they have a distorted view of drinking. There are plenty of people in the world, nondrinkers and ex-drinkers alike, who have no desire to drink. You were one of them once.

We are not born with the desire to drink. It is created by a combination of brainwashing and addiction and it can be easily removed. All you have to do is follow the instructions.

ALCOHOL IN FOCUS

By the time you finish reading this book your frame of mind will be such that, whenever you think about drinking, instead of feeling deprived because you can no longer drink, you will feel overjoyed because you no longer have to.

You will see alcohol for what it really is, just as you may see a drug like heroin now. It's easy for us to recognize the heroin trap. The things we are told about heroin as we are growing up are quite clear: ADDICTION! SLAVERY! POVERTY! MISERY! DEGRADATION! DEATH!

But alcohol is portrayed in a very different light.

We're not shown the desperate addicts dying of liver disease or homeless because they've squandered everything on booze; we're shown happy, beautiful people having fun or acting cool, showing no signs of strain or anxiety, enjoying all the pleasures that life has to offer. The message is straightforward: "Alcohol makes you happy."

But you know that's not the case, which is why you're reading this book. You have seen firsthand the harm that alcohol causes, so it's time to blow away the illusions once and for all, stop seeing drinking as a pleasure or crutch, and focus on the true picture.

If you can look at a heroin addict and see the mistake she's making when she thinks the next fix will make everything all right, you are already on the way to solving your own problem. The aim of this book is to help you find the happiness that comes with being free from the slavery of addiction. You'll see clearly that drinking does not relieve your misery at all; it is the cause of it. The alcohol trap is not a prison from which you can never escape; escape is easy provided you follow the right method. You have every reason to feel excited.

When you chose to read this book you made a statement that you have had enough of the alcohol trap. Perhaps you reached that point a long time ago but had no idea how to escape. You want to stop drinking and start living without feeling like a slave, but you don't want to spend the rest of your life feeling deprived. This book has all the instructions you need, so start looking forward to your great achievement and cast off any sense of doom and gloom.

THIRD INSTRUCTION:
START WITH A FEELING OF ELATION

Put the idea that stopping will be hard and painful out of your mind. It's a myth. Instead, look forward to a life free from alcohol.

Imagine how good you'll feel both physically and mentally. Think about the money you'll save and the joy you'll share with your friends and family. Most of all, think about the freedom without alcohol forever casting a shadow over your life. Feel the excitement growing as that freedom draws nearer. Nothing stands in your way now. Just keep following the instructions and your escape is guaranteed. You have nothing to lose and everything to gain.

SUMMARY

- **The first step to freedom is recognizing your problem as addiction, not just a habit you can't break**

- **Your addiction is not a weakness in you, nor something magical in the alcohol. It is a trap**

- **In order to escape permanently, you must remove the desire to drink**

- **The alcohol trap is the same as the heroin trap**

- **See alcohol in its true light and you will remove the desire**

- **Rejoice! Nothing stands in your way now**

- **THIRD INSTRUCTION: START WITH A FEELING OF ELATION**

Chapter 6

THE INCREDIBLE MACHINE

Your body is designed with all it needs to ensure your well-being and survival, but we tend to disregard the instincts that protect us from harm.

There are three powerful pieces of brainwashing that lead us into the alcohol trap:

1. The myth that the human mind and body are weak and need outside help in order to enjoy life and cope with stress.

2. The myth that alcohol will compensate for these illusory weaknesses.

3. The myth that humans are more intelligent than the intelligence that created us, whatever you believe that to be.

The belief that we are weak and incomplete creates our desire for alcohol, and the illusion that alcohol compensates for our weakness makes us feel dependent on it. It's a classic con trick, like selling a crutch riddled with woodworm to someone who doesn't have a broken leg.

Modern computers are incredible machines. There is seemingly no limit to the functions they can perform in the blink of an eye, but spill a glass of wine over your keyboard and that incredible machine suddenly becomes rather useless.

Now consider your body. That too is an incredible machine. Far more incredible than any computer. It can perform millions of functions all at the same time without you even initiating them or even being aware of them. What's more, you can pour wine into it for years and not only will it keep functioning, it might not even need to go in for repairs. That's if you're lucky. Not everyone is. But your body's ability to recover from the abuse you put it through is so remarkable it puts any industrial machine to shame.

Your body is incredibly strong and so are you. It is also incredibly sophisticated, capable of producing every chemical and every instinctive reaction it needs to survive. It boasts an early warning system designed to send you a clear signal when something is wrong. That signal is pain. But instead of regarding pain as a valuable survival facility, we treat it as an unnecessary evil and take drugs to anesthetize it. That's like stopping your smoke alarm from sounding by unplugging it instead of finding the fire and putting it out.

Your senses are also part of that early warning system. Sight, smell, touch, and taste all play a part in detecting poison. Watch an animal approach food. First they will look at it from a safe distance, then they will go up and sniff it. They might prod it with a paw and then, if all these senses are satisfied, they will taste it, tentatively at first.

Your senses do the same for you. You can tell when an apple is rotten by looking at it. If it's just overripe, it might look edible, but it will smell nasty and will be soft to the touch. If you took a bite, the taste would be repugnant and you would spit it out. An experience like that might put you off apples for life. There are no role models or friends pressurizing you to persevere.

Your senses are trying to protect you when you first drink alcohol. It might be designed to look appealing, but the smell is your first warning. The taste is your second. That first taste of alcohol repulses many. If you manage to get it down, the chances are you'll feel unpleasant or even ill. This is the next line of defense as your body does everything it can to expel the poison.

The coordination required to drive a car is incredible. Every second your brain manages a complex system of messages that come from your eyes and ears and are relayed to your hands and feet. You can steer, control your speed, change gear, check what's around you, talk to your passengers, change stations on the radio, and eat a snack all at the same time without ever coming close to causing an accident. But add alcohol and suddenly all this incredible coordination gets knocked out. People who drive under the influence of alcohol struggle to steer straight, let alone perform any other function.

Women and Wine

The problem of women's increasing wine consumption is hidden behind a jokey façade. For example, hundreds of thousands of women regularly take to "Moms Who Need Wine" or "OMG, I So Need A Glass of Wine or I'm Gonna Sell My Kids!" on Facebook, and wines marketed for women often have "amusing" labels such as "Girls Night Out," "Cupcake," or "Mommy's Time Out." There are refrigerator magnets and dish towels that say things like "All you need is love and a glass of wine" or "Home is where the wine is waiting." A big joke is always made out of the situation.

Popular TV programs don't always help either. For example, female characters in sitcoms regularly open bottles of wine whenever there is a crisis... as if it will really help. In the U.S.A., so much wine is drunk by characters in *The Real Housewives* series that several actresses have developed lucrative sidelines fronting up their own wine brands.

The result is that wine is now mistakenly seen as stress relief for women, and each year it seems to come in bigger and bigger glasses.

In fact, women consume the lion's share of the 800 gallons bought annually in the U.S.A.; in 2013 out of $21.2 billion spent on wine, women accounted for 59 percent of consumption.

It's all heading out of control. A recent study of binge drinking—defined as four or more drinks for women in two hours—conducted by Centers for Disease Control and Prevention found that 10 percent of U.S. women between 45 and 64 admitted they binge drink, and so did 3 percent of over-65s.

THE FLAW IN THE INCREDIBLE MACHINE

The human body is anything but weak and deficient, yet we suffer in ways that the rest of the animal kingdom do not. You don't see wild animals destroying themselves with drug addiction and suffering bouts of self-loathing, so how come humankind, the most intelligent species on the planet, falls victim to self-inflicted ailments time and time again?

The clue lies in that word "intelligent." The vital difference between human beings and wild animals is that animals survive solely by instinct. Humans also use instinct to survive, but the tool that has enabled us to rule over the animal kingdom is intellect.

Our intellect has given us the capacity to learn and pass on our learning, with the result that we have developed into a highly sophisticated species that is not only capable of building fantastic structures and machines but also has an appreciation of art, music, romance, spirituality, and so on. Intellect is a wonderful thing, but it can go to your head; for it is our intellect that has also led us astray.

Look again at the "advances" humankind has made and

you'll see that, rather than building on the advantage that Mother Nature has given us, we have devoted a remarkable amount of time to self-destruction – not just in the ever-more-sophisticated ways of killing each other we've developed, but even in the food we eat. By allowing our intellect to override our instincts, we have become a species of compulsive junk food consumers.

SWEET NOTHING

Fruit is the food that nature designed us to eat above any other and our taste for the natural sugar in fruit is designed to keep us coming back for more. Refined sugar, packed into candy, cakes, and alcoholic drinks, is designed to replicate the sweetness of fruit. It contains none of the goodness of fruit, but it tricks our taste buds into thinking it's the same thing. Intellectually we have created a substance that fools our instincts into thinking we are getting something good when, in truth, it is nothing but bad.

Instinct is Mother Nature's survival kit. It tells us when and what to eat; it alerts us to danger; it even helps us to find a suitable mate. But there are times when it conflicts with our intellect and then we tend to trust the lessons we've learned over our instincts. Why? Because instinct often gives us the answer we don't want to hear.

The pain of childbirth happens for a reason. It triggers hormones that play a vital role before, during, and after delivery, such as helping to control the speed of the birth and helping the mother to bond with her baby. Pain-relieving drugs interfere with the production of these hormones.

But if a doctor comes in and offers you pain relief, you're likely to trust his advice over your own instincts. It is exactly this, our tendency to trust in intellectual opinion over and above our own instincts, that is the flaw that leads us into the alcohol trap. When we make intellectual choices based on misinformation—like drinking alcohol to help us relax—our well-being suffers. Wild animals do not experience bouts of self-loathing. Intellect causes misery just as it causes happiness. The choice is ours. So why do we so often take the self-destructive option? Quite simply,

WE DON'T ALWAYS REALIZE WE HAVE AN OPTION

There are always people who stand to gain as a result of these destructive human practices, be they drug dealers, the tobacco and alcoholic drinks industries, fast food chains, gambling firms, or whatever, and they have become expert at exploiting our intellect to hoodwink us into making misguided choices.

Nobody chooses to become a drinker for the rest of their life. We don't swallow that first drink thinking, "Great! I'm on my way to becoming an alcoholic." We swallow it because we think it is the thing to do.

Our instincts are screaming at us to stop, doing everything in their power to reject the poison, but we push through the pain barrier because we believe it's something we must do.

We are pressurized into drinking by society, by our peers, by our role models, and by our own beliefs, formed from years of brainwashing. In the face of such pressure, is it any wonder so many of us fall for the alcohol trap?

SEPARATING TRUTH FROM ILLUSION

The myth that drinking gives you pleasure or a crutch and the myth that stopping will be hard and painful are the two illusions that prevent addicts from escaping the trap. I've explained why so many people get taken in by these illusions, but another question may have crossed your mind:

How do I know that Easyway is not just conning me that they are illusions?

When you see through an illusion and recognize the truth, you can never be fooled into buying into the illusion again. Even if you did get a genuine high each time you drank, would it be worth it for the low that follows, for the misery and self-loathing, the emotional and financial cost, the damage to your health, and relationships?

The fact is the illusion of pleasure *is* an illusion and Easyway is *not* brainwashing. It's fact, but don't just take our word for it; you can tell for yourself. If you want to check just how easy it is to trick the human mind, have a look again at the table illusion in Chapter Two (page 44).

There's another illusion coming up on the next page to emphasize the point.

Above are some irregular black shapes. Do you see a message? At first, it might look like a random line of building blocks. If so, look again. This time look at the shapes with your eyes half closed (through your eyelashes) and you can make a word appear. It might help if you move your head back a little (or to one side) and look again from a distance. You should see the word "STOP."

The word hasn't suddenly appeared; it's been there all along. If you couldn't see it that's because you thought you were looking at an irregular black shape. After all, that is what you were told. So you were focusing on the black rather than the shapes around it.

Once you can see the word STOP, it becomes almost impossible to look at the pattern and not see it. But until you're told it's there, you could very well never find it. But there is a much clearer message and once you see it you will always see it. The same is true of any argument. If you are only shown one side, you will have no reason to doubt it. Only when you are shown both sides do you have a choice as to which you believe. And once you've seen the truth, you can never be fooled again.

This graphic deliberately misleads you, just as the alcoholic drinks industry deliberately misleads you into believing that alcohol gives you some sort of pleasure or crutch. The medical profession and other help organizations actually support this one-sided view. Only Easyway points out the alternative: that alcohol does absolutely nothing for you whatsoever. When you start to examine this side of the argument, you quickly see that it is true and you can never again be fooled into believing the opposite.

You fell into the alcohol trap because you were under the illusion that drinking gave you pleasure and/or a crutch. And yet drinking has not made you happy and secure; it has made you miserable and afraid. The truth is plain to see and now that you've seen it, nothing will be able to change your perception.

So let's take a closer look at those illusions.

SUMMARY

• **The human body and mind are incredibly strong and do not need outside help**

• **We come unstuck when we allow our intellect to override our instincts**

• **Once you see both sides of an argument, you can choose which one to believe. If you only see one side, you are being brainwashed**

• **Once you see the truth, you can never be fooled again**

Chapter 7

THE ILLUSIONS

IN THIS CHAPTER
•IT TASTES GREAT •PARTY TIME •LOSS OF JUDGMENT
•TIME TO UNWIND •IT'S JUST A HABIT
•IT'S THE WAY I'M MADE •DENIAL

It's time to take a new look at all the illusions that contribute to the alcohol trap and see the real picture.

IT TASTES GREAT

If you need reminding how alcoholic drinks really taste, think back to the first time you tried one. Can you honestly say that the first time you tasted vodka, or gin, or wine, or any other alcoholic drink, you thought it tasted delicious? Wasn't it, in fact, repulsive? Wasn't your immediate instinct to gag, or convulse, or spit it out?

If you ever tasted neat alcohol you would understand why. It's not advisable. Neat alcohol is pure poison and a half pint of it is enough to kill you. Yet the alcoholic drinks industry has succeeded in convincing most of the world that its product tastes great—a classic case of intellect overriding instinct.

We've explained how our senses are designed to protect us and help us to survive. When it comes to drinking, our taste buds are designed to find the best thing we can to quench our thirst:

water. Water is an important nutrient and we cannot survive without it for more than a couple of days. Imagine you'd been two days walking across the desert and you finally arrived at a bar. They offered you a glass of water or a glass of wine. Which would you take?

You might be one of those people who wants nothing more on a hot day than a cold, thirst-quenching glass of rosé or beer. If that drink seems thirst-quenching it's because it's 95 percent water. Your thirst would be better quenched by a glass of pure water, but there's something more than thirst making you crave that glass of beer or rosé: your craving for alcohol. So when you drink it, you're not only relieving your thirst, you're relieving an alcohol craving too.

Alcohol is not thirst-quenching at all. It is a diuretic, which means it dehydrates you; therefore, it works against the thirst-quenching effects of the water and leaves you wanting more. That's why people manage to drink such large quantities of alcohol in a single evening. You couldn't do that with water; your thirst would be quickly satisfied.

The drinks manufacturers mask the poisonous taste of alcohol with natural flavors: hops, grapes, juniper, orange, lemon, lime, raspberry... the flavors of fruit—the flavors we were designed by nature to enjoy. Fruit gives us vital nutrients too. So if, once you've acquired the loss of taste necessary to drink alcohol without revulsion, you develop an appreciation of the subtler flavors of wine, say, it has nothing to do with the alcohol and everything to do with the fruit.

In which case shouldn't soft drinks give us the same satisfaction?

Who's saying they don't? Perhaps you've tried spending an evening in a bar drinking soft drinks and found it anything but satisfying, but think back to that bar in the desert: When your mouth is parched after two days without water, a soft drink is much more satisfying than an alcoholic one. It's only when you're programmed to expect alcohol—in a bar, out to dinner, at a party —that soft drinks don't satisfy.

Can you see through the illusion now? The truth is clear: It is your craving for alcohol that makes you drink booze in these situations. It has nothing to do with the taste.

DRINKING IS FUN!

We become programmed to expect alcohol in certain situations because of another popular myth: that drinking helps to make social occasions more enjoyable. This is based on two further illusions:

1. The illusion that alcohol gives you courage.

2. The illusion that alcohol makes you more entertaining.

Some social occasions can be daunting. We worry about having to meet new people. Will we get on? Will we have anything interesting to say? We reach for our little crutch to quell these fears and, lo and behold, we find we feel a little less intimidated and awkward when we walk into the crowd. But how does this actually affect our enjoyment of the situation?

The term "Dutch courage" originates from a time in history when British troops fighting France's Louis XIV alongside their allies from the Low Countries (the Netherlands) appreciated the seemingly calming effects of Jenever (Dutch gin) before heading into battle. How did it work? By numbing the instinct of fear. There is a difference between being fearless and being courageous. Courage is acting in spite of fear. Think of the amazing men and women of the fire service. A firefighter who runs into a burning building to rescue a baby is not fearless; she knows the danger she is in and her heart will be pounding, but she sets her fear aside to save the life of the baby. That is courage.

Take away the fear with alcohol and you might well run into that burning building, but the chances of you running out again are slim. Fear serves a vital purpose in our survival. It is the emotion that saves us from danger by triggering the "fight or flight" response. When we are threatened, we need all our faculties to be fully functional: the ability to run, to shout, to fight, to think. Fear triggers all these responses. Knock out fear with alcohol and you are effectively burying your head in the sand. The effect is twofold and fatal: you not only fail to

> *"One reason I don't drink is that I want to know when I am having a good time."*
> **Lady Astor**
> (who in 1919 became the first woman to sit as a Member of Parliament [MP] in the U.K. House of Commons)

identify danger when it arises, you also lack the ability to respond.

A party is not a life or death situation, so you might ask what does it matter if you knock out your fears rather than overcoming them with courage? Apart from the fact that there *are* dangers associated with some social occasions, especially for women, nullifying your fears with alcohol is like removing the bulb from the oil warning light in your car. You never tackle the root of the problem and so it never goes away. In fact, it guarantees that it will get worse.

Think about the fears that make you feel inhibited: meeting new people, finding things to say, looking your best, being liked… All these challenges are within your control. You can influence how you come across in social situations by preparing yourself mentally. The more you practice the better you get, but if you always bury your head in the sand and avoid these challenges, you will never learn to cope. Moreover,

THE MORE YOU DRINK, THE LESS CONTROL YOU HAVE OVER HOW YOU COME ACROSS

Therefore, alcohol actually reduces your ability to enjoy social occasions to the full. Not only does it knock out your fears, it knocks out your judgment, your ability to react and respond, and ultimately your control over your actions and words.

Far from making you more entertaining, it makes you dull or even offensive and embarrassing company and leaves you with a blank, meaningless experience—often followed by days of feeling intensely foolish, self-loathing and regretful.

Perhaps you are shy and don't enjoy having to talk about yourself or find it difficult to talk to people you don't know. But think about it, who would you rather spend time talking to— someone who doesn't talk much but listens, or someone who talks too much and shows no interest in what you have to say? Shyness is an incredibly attractive and enchanting trait. Social convention makes the shy person feel vulnerable in unfamiliar company, but any sense of inadequacy is only in their own mind. Brash, talkative people hog the limelight and thus create the false impression that they are more entertaining and interesting than everyone else, but in fact most people are secretly wishing they would shut up and give someone else the floor.

ALCOHOL DOESN'T MAKE US MORE INTERESTING; IT JUST REMOVES OUR ABILITY TO TELL WHEN WE'RE BEING DULL, RUDE, OR OBNOXIOUS

Try to drown your shyness with booze and you increase the likelihood of making a fool of yourself. Good manners are also a form of inhibition: We employ tact to control our thoughts about someone so as not to hurt their feelings or cause antagonism. Drunks often become rude and abusive because they override their normal sense of tact. They also become aggressive and accuse people of being rude to them. What fun is that? Perhaps at this very moment, you are trying to block your mind to such events in your recent past. Don't panic—just think how wonderful it will be to be free.

TAKE CARE

Making a fool of yourself or being rude to people is unattractive, but there are other inhibitions that, when knocked out, can lead to far more serious consequences. A woman who goes home with a stranger at the end of the evening is putting herself in a vulnerable situation. If she's sober, she will be acutely aware of the risks involved and will be better able to judge the stranger's character and intentions. Drunk, her reading of the situation is impaired and she puts herself in danger.

We are equipped with many social skills designed to help maintain a civilized society: politeness, tolerance, tact, diplomacy, the ability to listen, the ability to show an interest in others, the ability to pacify. Alcohol knocks out all these skills and the results are what we regard as stereotypical drunken behavior:

Insensitivity

Long-windedness

Rudeness

Impatience

Abusiveness

Boorishness

Aggression

Violence

Indiscretion

Poor judgment

The inability to know when to stop can have deadly consequences. It's very rare for two sober people to come to blows. In most confrontations, there's a lot of talk

> *"When you go out with a drunk, you'll notice how a drunk fills your glass so he can empty his own. As long as you're drinking, drinking is okay. Two's company… If there's a bottle, even if your glass isn't empty, he'll pour a little in your glass before he fills his own."*
> **Chuck Palahniuk**

and posturing as both parties go through the primitive ritual of trying to face their opponent down. Neither one wants to hit or be hit, and in most cases they will back down before it comes to that. But add alcohol to the mix and the sense that inhibits violence is knocked out. The primitive instincts that enable us to assess the situation and weigh up our chances of emerging unscathed —or, indeed, inflicting grievous harm—stop working. It's no surprise that the increase in women drinking has coincided with an increase in violence among women.

Perhaps you think this is an extreme picture—most social occasions pass off without anyone being seriously hurt in a drunken fight. Extreme as these examples are, they are by no means uncommon. The simple truth is

ALCOHOL DOESN'T GIVE YOU ANY POWERS; IT TAKES YOUR POWERS AWAY

The misconception that alcohol is necessary for having a good time leads many people to spoil the occasion and have a bad time. Once you've freed yourself from alcohol and learned once again to trust in your ability to get on with other people and have fun, just as we do as children, you will go into all social occasions with greater confidence and come out having had more fun than ever. It's not about having some sort of puritanical lifestyle—it's extraordinary, but every aspect of every physical experience is enhanced and heightened by sobriety.

IT RELAXES ME

You come home after a long, hard day, kick off your shoes, flop into an armchair and sigh, "I could murder a drink." You're stressed, your nerves are frayed, and you believe that alcohol will help you unwind. You've seen the same scene acted out countless times on TV and in movies. Everybody knows that a good stiff drink will help you to relax, don't they?

In fact, the opposite is true.

Just like fear, nerves and stress serve an important purpose. They alert us to threats. That threat might be simply that you're overdoing it and need to give your

> *"Alcoholism is a devastating, potentially fatal disease. The primary symptom of having it is telling everyone —including yourself—that you are not an alcoholic."*
>
> Herbert L. Gravitz
> and Julie D. Bowden

mind and body a rest. As I've already mentioned, by numbing the sensation with alcohol, all you're doing is removing the warning light instead of resolving the problem. And if the problem is left to get worse, the stress will increase.

Alcohol is also a major cause of stress. The restless feeling it creates as it leaves your system will make you feel stressed and nervous until you satisfy it. But remember what you've learned about the nature of addiction: You can never completely relieve that restless feeling it creates. The only way to do that is to become a nondrinker.

Drinking alcohol to relieve the stress caused by drinking alcohol is as illogical as wearing tight shoes just for the pleasure of taking them off!

On average, one unit of alcohol is metabolized in one hour. So after just one hour any relaxing effect the alcohol had will have worn off, the stress will have returned, and with it the new stress caused by the drink. In other words, the more you drink, the more stressed you become. So much for it helping you to relax,

ALCOHOL PREVENTS YOU FROM UNWINDING

The best treatment for stress is sleep and, as every drinker knows, alcohol impairs sleep. When you get home from a long, hard day, kick off your shoes, take a shower, change your clothes, eat something, flop in your armchair… all these actions will help you to relax and relieve stress, but all the good will be undone if you drink alcohol.

IT'S JUST A HABIT

People frequently use the word "habit" when talking about addiction. They talk about someone having a "drug habit," as if it's just a thing they do like putting their car keys in a particular place when they get home. But there is a clear distinction between habit and addiction, and it's important that you understand what it is if you are to grasp the nature of the victim and the trap.

With habits, you are in control. They might be pleasant or unpleasant habits, but you follow them only because you want to. If you had to stop them, you could do so easily and immediately. An addiction is a repeated action that you wish you didn't do but can't stop, or wish you did less but can't.

You might believe that you choose to drink because it gives you some sort of pleasure or crutch, but take your head out of the sand and list all the advantages and disadvantages of drinking alcohol, and you would have to conclude that there is no sense in it whatsoever.

This is why all drinkers (and all other addicts) instinctively feel stupid. But it's not stupidity at all. How can it be stupid if you're not the one controlling it?

> *"One key symptom of alcoholism is that the individual comes to need a drink for every mood—one to calm down, one to perk up, one to celebrate, one to deal with disappointment, and so on."*
>
> Phyllis A. Balch

Calling your drinking a habit is effectively saying, "I don't understand why I do it. I don't get any genuine pleasure from it." So why not stop? Because there is a powerful force compelling you to carry on. Only by recognizing that force as addiction and understanding how it works will you be able to free yourself forever.

That doesn't mean you will resist the temptation; it means there will be no temptation. You will have no need or desire to drink.

IT'S THE WAY I'M MADE

By dismissing your drinking as "just a habit," you attempt to shirk responsibility for dealing with it. The same is true of drinkers who claim it's just the way they're made. They put their failure to quit down to one of two things:

1. A weakness in their temperament—a lack of willpower.

2. A predisposition to alcoholism or addiction, over which they have no control—an addictive personality or a genetic predisposition.

Both excuses are a cop-out, blaming something that cannot be changed and thus giving themselves a license to continue doing it, or getting some kind of comfort from their feeling of hopelessness that surrounds their repeated failed attempts to quit.

It suits the drinker who's afraid of quitting to believe they have a flaw in their nature that prevents them from being free because it enables them to avoid facing up to their problem and doing something about it. But the danger will not go away and neither will the fear and misery of being in the alcohol trap.

To convince them otherwise we have to overcome the weight of popular opinion that you *do* need willpower to quit, that there *is* such a thing as an addictive personality, and that if some kind of genetic predisposition does exist that it somehow inhibits escape from addiction.

This misinformation is put about by reputable organizations, so it's natural that millions of people should believe it, but it's as damaging to your chances of escape as the alcohol itself. Why would an organization that genuinely wants to help people stop drinking spread a belief that serves to imprison them more deeply in the trap? Simply because they too have been brainwashed and have never stopped to look at the situation another way.

Remember the STOP illusion. Once you look at it in a different way and see the true message, you can never be fooled by the illusion again.

That's why it's essential that you keep an open mind and follow all the instructions in order: because the truth is often the complete opposite of what you've been told.

All drinkers, like all addicts, lie. They lie to themselves and to others. Not because they're bad people—it's simply what addiction does. We're constantly looking for any excuse to justify our behavior.

"It gives me a buzz"—"it relaxes me."

"It makes life fun"—"it's just a habit."

All these excuses amount to one thing: ***DENIAL***

Instead of truth and freedom, the addict in denial opts for lies and imprisonment. It's an illogical choice, but it's one that millions of people make every day. Like the ostrich that buries its head in the sand, they think they can cocoon themselves from their fears by blinding themselves to them. So what are drinkers really afraid of? It's time we looked more closely at your fears.

SUMMARY

- You don't acquire a taste for alcohol; you acquire a loss of taste
- Alcohol doesn't give you any powers; it takes your powers away
- Alcohol makes you more stressed and fearful
- Drinking is not a habit; it's an addiction
- You get hooked on drink because you have taken an addictive drug, not because of any flaw in your personality or because of any genetic predisposition
- All excuses for drinking are just a form of denial

Chapter 8

FEAR

The brainwashing creates a tug of war of conflicting fears that form a barrier to quitting. This requires us to remove some more of the brainwashing.

All drinkers are constantly plagued by contradictions. They are aware of the misery that drinking is causing them and of the terrible risk they run of destroying their health, wealth, and relationships, yet they also believe that alcohol provides them with some sort of pleasure or crutch.

Lots of double standards operate against women in society, including the pressures on them to drink, and also not to drink. Women who come to Easyway centers often do so because, for a variety of reasons, they have been advised by their doctor to stop drinking. Women actually tend to heed this advice more than men. Women also confide that they do a lot of things they regret under the influence of alcohol. They tend not to be able to laugh them off like men do.

Binge drinking, as women at our centers frequently tell us, can lead to one or all of the following:

- a deep sense of shame and paranoia

- blackouts and anxiety about not knowing what has happened under the influence of alcohol

- terrible hangovers

- ill-advised one-night stands

- drink-driving

- a deep feeling of having made a fool of yourself

- regrets at taking absurd risks that could have endangered individual or family happiness (and which they would never take if sober)

- unhappiness at having to conceal what they have done, and how much they drink, from other members of the family

- arguments and violence

- the deterioration of looks caused by too much drinking

• disruption of home life and embarrassment at work

• depression

There are so many reasons to stop drinking, yet women make excuses that enable them to go on because they are afraid of what might happen if they try to quit. They fear life without their little crutch. If you believe all the myths and illusions about drinking— that it tastes great, that it makes social occasions more enjoyable, that it relaxes you and gives you courage—it follows that you believe that life will be empty, difficult, or even impossible without it.

All drinkers find themselves in a tug of war of fear: afraid to go on drinking and afraid to quit.

"I know it's going to ruin me, but it's my one pleasure in life."

"I'm afraid of losing my family, but I can't imagine coping with life or enjoying life without booze."

As we explained in the last chapter, fear is designed to protect us. We shouldn't treat it as a negative. It is the instinct that protects us from real dangers—but fear is also our response to imaginary dangers too. Our intellect has enabled us to learn about potential dangers and how to avoid them, so much so that we can be fearful of dangers that don't exist.

For example, you can fear the prospect of losing all your money. You may have no experience of having no money, nor be in any immediate danger of it, yet you can imagine what it would be like because you have learned about it. This is an intellectual fear. You can be in no actual danger of becoming destitute and know you are in no danger, yet still fear it. There are millionaires who live in fear of poverty. That's probably why they're millionaires—they do everything in their power to safeguard their money.

The fear of losing everything enables the millionaire to guard against it, but what if your projected fears are based on false information? Say, for example, you read that fruit causes cancer. You would probably avoid eating fruit. You would also worry about the damage already done by all the fruit you've eaten in your life. As consumers, it's impossible for us to know what to believe and we spend a lot of our life worrying about things that will never happen. When we try to set aside our fears, we often become blasé about genuine dangers, such is the confusion from the mixed messages we receive.

There are two types of fear that keep us from trying to escape.

FEAR OF FAILURE

The alcohol trap feels like a prison. Every aspect of your life is controlled by drinking: your daily routine, your view of the future, your suffering. The prison is in your mind, but it keeps you trapped just as securely as a physical prison and as long as you remain a slave to alcohol you will experience the same psychological symptoms as an inmate in a physical prison.

Anyone who has tried to quit and failed will know that it leaves you feeling more firmly trapped than you did before. You've seen movies where a woman is thrown into a room and the door locked behind her. The first thing she does is run to the door and wrench at the handle. This confirms her predicament: She really is locked in and her panic becomes worse and she eventually retreats, resigned to her fate. Trying and failing to quit has the same effect on the drinker. It reinforces the belief that you are trapped in a prison from which there is no escape.

This can be a crushing experience. Whereas once you might have told yourself you will quit one day, just not yet, now you are faced with the grim realization that you can't kid yourself any more. Many addicts conclude that the best way to avoid this misery is to avoid trying to quit in the first place. As long as they never try to escape, they will always preserve the belief that escape is possible. It is only when they try to escape that they have to admit it's impossible.

This is the twisted logic of addiction and you can see how self-defeating it is, yet there are millions of intelligent people who continue to delude themselves in this way. They prefer to continue suffering the misery of addiction than risk the misery of failure. What they don't realize is:

THE DOOR ONLY REMAINS SHUT IF YOU USE THE WRONG METHOD TO OPEN IT

Imagine your burning ambition was to be a dancer, but you were afraid of being rejected so you never went to auditions. What would be your chances of becoming a dancer? Zero. By protecting yourself from the fear of failure, you guarantee that you fail.

With drink, the fear of failure is the fear of remaining a drinker. But you're already a drinker, so you're fearing something that has already happened. If you continue to avoid even trying to escape, you guarantee that you will feel a failure for the rest of your life.

For the dancer who does attend the audition, fear of failure is a positive force. It focuses her mind, drives her to practice harder, and gives her an energy that is compelling to watch. The same is true for all of us: When channeled positively, the fear of failure can magnify our abilities.

By trying to quit drinking, you give yourself a chance of success. By trying to quit with Easyway, you give yourself the best possible chance. By following all the instructions in order, from beginning to end, you cannot fail.

IF YOU SUCCUMB TO THE FEAR OF FAILURE, YOU ARE GUARANTEED TO FAIL

FEAR OF SUCCESS

We can all understand the misery of being in prison and find it hard to understand why anyone who has spent time in one would reoffend after being released, thus running the risk of going back in. Yet this happens with depressing regularity, particularly among prisoners who have spent a long time behind bars. We assume it's because they haven't learned the error of their ways, but often it's because they actually *want* to go back inside. They yearn for the "security" of the prison.

Life on the outside is alien and frightening for them: It doesn't run to the same routine or the same guidelines; it's not what they know and they don't feel equipped to handle it.

For addicts, life without their little crutch is also frightening. They don't know how they'll cope without it; they think they'll have to go through some terrible trauma to get free and that they'll be condemned to a life of sacrifice and deprivation.

We're tricked into believing that life without drinking is boring and stressful. Though you're well aware of the misery that drinking causes, you may have come to regard it as part of your identity. The Hollywood image of the heavy drinker, the chain smoker, and the gambler can suggest that it makes us attractive. Heroic characters in books and movies are frequently portrayed as having one or more of these characteristics and the implication is that it makes them human, charming, exciting, lovable. To the audience maybe—in real life it makes them miserable and impossible to live with.

The fear of success is based on the illusions that we have already dealt with. If you have followed all the instructions and understood everything you've read so far, you will know that drinking does absolutely nothing for you and so there is nothing to lose when you stop. On the contrary, you will make many wonderful gains—one of which is no longer having to live in fear.

WIN THE TUG OF WAR

Fear lies at the root of all addictions. It is the force that makes the trap so ingenious because it works back to front. It's when you are not drinking that you suffer the empty, insecure feeling. When you drink, you feel a small boost, which partially relieves the insecurity, and your brain is fooled into believing that the alcohol is providing a crutch. In fact, it is alcohol that created the fear. The more you drink, the more it drags you down and the greater your need for the crutch.

This is why you can never win while you're in the trap. When you can't drink, you wish you could; when you're drinking, you wish you didn't have to. The tug of war of fear becomes easy to win when you see that the fears pulling you from both sides are caused by the same thing: alcohol.

TAKE AWAY THE ALCOHOL AND THE FEAR GOES TOO

If you don't drink, you can't fear the consequences of drinking. At the same time, you open your eyes to the truth about life without drinking. If you could feel now what you will feel when you finish the book and quit, you would wonder, "Will I really feel this good?" Fear will have been replaced by elation, despair by optimism, self-doubt by confidence, apathy by energy. Your physical health will improve, you will feel full of life, and you will find it much easier to relax.

If you've quit in the past but not felt as good as this, it's because you were having to use willpower. Somewhere in your mind you still believed you were making a sacrifice and so you never really freed yourself of the misery. With Easyway, you will not miss drink at all. You will remove all desire to drink and it will be clear in your mind that you are not giving anything up. All you are doing is removing something from your life that has made you miserable and replacing it with something that makes you genuinely happy: freedom.

THERE IS NOTHING TO FEAR

Get it clearly into your mind that alcohol is your worst enemy and, far from giving you pleasure or a crutch, it's driving you deeper and deeper into misery and despair. Isn't that why you're reading this book? You instinctively know this, so open your mind and follow your instincts.

REMOVE ALL DOUBTS

Make a list of everything you stand to gain by breaking free from the alcohol trap. Your self-respect will soar now that you're no longer having to cover up, lie to your friends and family, deceive your workmates, and convince yourself that you are in control. You'll have more time and more money and you'll feel fantastic. That little boost you feel every time you satisfy your craving for drink is a mere hint of how a nondrinker feels all the time and how you will feel too when you're free. Wouldn't you rather feel like that all the time, without any effort or cost, and without the horrible lows that alcohol brings?

You have every reason to quit drinking and no reason to continue. There is nothing to fear in quitting, only marvelous gains to look forward to. Wouldn't you say the same if you met a heroin addict? Wouldn't you point out that the "high" she thinks she gets from the drug is nothing more than relief from the terrible craving caused by the drug leaving her body, and that the only way to relieve it completely and permanently is to stop taking the drug? Perhaps you don't see the comparison between yourself and a heroin addict. Believe it, all addicts are the same. The trap works in exactly the same way and the solution for you is just as simple.

The only reason you might fail to see the solution as simple is because you have been brainwashed into the tug of war of fear. Once you can see that there is nothing to fear, that you are not giving up anything or depriving yourself in any way, stopping is easy.

It's essential that you get it clear in your mind that drinking does absolutely nothing positive for you whatsoever, that the beliefs that have imprisoned you in the alcohol trap are merely illusions, and that you have everything to gain and nothing to lose by stopping. If you have any lingering doubts, we must remove them now. Go back and read the last two chapters again if you are unclear on any of the arguments about the illusions that create the fear that underlies all addictions. You need to be fully prepared for the next instruction.

FOURTH INSTRUCTION:
NEVER DOUBT YOUR DECISION TO QUIT

You have picked up this book because you want to cure your alcohol addiction. You have come a long way in the process already and you have the same chance of success as all the millions of people who have already quit with Easyway. Always remember your reasons for wanting to quit and never let doubt creep into your mind.

Sometimes people say they understand all the instructions, yet they still have doubts about the method. They haven't yet removed all the brainwashing and they still find it hard to believe they can quit without using willpower. It's time to unravel the willpower myth once and for all.

SUMMARY

- **Drinkers are pulled in two directions by a tug of war of fear**
- **Succumb to the fear of failure and you guarantee failure**
- **The fear of success is based on illusions**
- **Remove alcohol and you remove the fear**
- **Open your mind to the marvelous gains of ending your drinking problem. There is nothing to fear**
- **FOURTH INSTRUCTION: NEVER DOUBT YOUR DECISION TO QUIT**

Chapter 9

WILLPOWER

If you think you have failed to quit drinking because you lack the willpower, think again. The willpower method is more likely to make your problems worse.

Most drinkers believe that stopping is hard. They also believe that you can't stop without willpower. So they try to stop by applying all their willpower and find it's incredibly hard. They conclude that they lack the necessary willpower to overcome the difficulty and quit trying.

But look at the situation another way. If drinkers who find it hard to stop are using willpower, doesn't that suggest that it's the use of willpower that makes it hard?

It's not the drinkers' fault that they don't make this connection. All the received wisdom from governments and health organizations is that you need willpower to quit. Only Easyway takes the opposite view. Only Easyway shows it exactly how it is.

People who try to quit with the willpower method never win

the tug of war of fear. On one side their rational brain knows they should stop drinking because it's making them ill, affecting their behavior, costing them a fortune, controlling their life, and causing misery. On the other side their addicted brain makes them panic at the thought of being deprived of their little crutch. It's this conflict that makes it hard to quit. Whether you drink or not, you are guaranteed to remain miserable. When you're not drinking you feel deprived and when you do drink you wish you didn't have to.

The willpower method requires you to focus on all the reasons for stopping and hope you can last long enough without drinking for the desire to eventually go. But as long as you continue to believe that drinking gives you pleasure or a crutch, the desire will never go.

When you remove the desire to drink, quitting is as easy as pushing open a door. But if you've ever come across a door with no handle and pushed on the wrong side, where the hinges are, you'll know how even the simplest of tasks can be hard if you go about it in the wrong way. The door might budge a tiny bit, but it won't swing open. It requires a huge amount of effort and determination. Push on the correct side and the door opens without you even having to think about it.

ENCOURAGING SOMEONE TO QUIT THROUGH THE USE OF WILLPOWER IS LIKE TELLING THEM TO OPEN A DOOR BY PUSHING ON THE HINGES

You only need willpower to stop drinking if you have a conflict of will. Our aim is to resolve that conflict by removing one side of the tug of war, so that you have no desire to drink.

HOW WEAK-WILLED ARE YOU?

When women drinkers try and fail to quit with the willpower method, rather than blame the method they tend to blame themselves. They assume that they are weak-willed. If you think you're unable to quit because you lack the necessary willpower, then you clearly don't understand the nature of the trap you're in.

Think how much willpower it took for you to overcome those first revolting drinks until you became immune to the taste. Is it not your will to keep drinking that has driven you to carry on in the face of overwhelming arguments to quit, and indeed your own desire to quit? There is plenty of evidence to suggest that problem drinkers are actually strong-willed, not weak-willed.

Many drinkers are also smokers, gamblers, and overeaters. You might interpret this as further evidence of a weak will. You just can't resist temptation. But temptation is the desire to do something you really enjoy. You don't enjoy drinking; it makes you miserable. The same is true of smoking, gambling, over-eating, and all other addictions. We wish we could stop but can't. The force that keeps you hooked is not temptation; it's addiction.

There is a connection between multiple addictions, but it's not that they are signs of a lack of willpower. On the contrary, they are more likely evidence of a strong will. What they all share is that they are traps created by brainwashing. And one of the biggest myths is that quitting requires willpower.

Decisions, Decisions

Modern women's lives are complex. You're making decisions not just for yourself but for others in the family too. On average, around 80 percent of household decisions are made by women: what food is bought, upkeep of the house, health, education, vacations, and even looking after cars. It's not easy. You're making decisions all the time, not just for you but for everyone else. You have to think of everything. This leads to pressure.

In an ever-changing world, women are taking on more and more roles and having to resolve competing demands: work versus home life; kids versus partner; what you need versus the needs of everybody else. The more you worry, the less you get done. Studies show that the worse women feel about drinking too much one evening, the more likely they are to overdo it on the evenings which follow. But you have to realize that drinking never helps you at all. In fact it never helps anyone. Making decisions and managing your life are much easier without alcohol.

IN HER OWN WORDS: RACHEL

As the manager of a sports center in the 1980s, I found myself having to fight my corner in a man's world. It could be quite pressurized at times, but I relished the challenge and enjoyed it when I got my way. To be honest, I got my way most of the time. I think some of the men I dealt with were scared of me! But we got on well and often went out drinking together, both for work and socially.

In my late 20s, I decided it was time to start a family and the first thing I needed to do was cut down on the drinking. I wanted to be in good health for my baby. I thought it would be easy, but as time went by and I couldn't get pregnant, I started to console myself with a drink in the evening. Pretty soon that became a drink or two at lunchtime and before long I was drinking as much as ever.

I went to see the doctor about my inability to get pregnant and she asked me how much I drank. I lied to her, but she was still surprised by my answer and told me I should try to stop. So I did. I tried with all my might, but although I had a very good reason for not drinking, I just couldn't get the craving for drink out of my mind. I found it really frustrating. I had never had a problem getting my way before and in every other facet of life, if I turned my mind to something I knew I could achieve it. But when it came to drink, I just seemed to be too weak-willed.

I wish I'd known then what I know now. Being weak-willed wasn't the problem; it was the belief that I was depriving myself of a genuine pleasure. Despite all the good reasons to stop, part of me didn't want to be dictated to in that way and so I kept drinking. It was my strength of will that kept me drinking!

It takes a strong will to persist in doing something that goes against all your instincts. When you organize your daily life so you can sneak to the stores to buy booze without arousing suspicion; when you get up early in the morning or stay up late at night so you can drink without your family looking over your shoulder; when you borrow money from friends and lie to them about what you need it for; when you sacrifice the pastimes you used to enjoy because your only interest in life is drink... all these things take a strong will.

The world is full of strong-willed people with alcohol problems. Famous sports stars, actors and actresses, singers, writers, politicians... the rehab centers are full of people who have found success and made a name for themselves in such fields. You don't get to the top of any industry if you're weak-willed. It takes determination, persistence, and hard work. So why would someone with the willpower to be the best in their field lack the willpower to quit drinking? The answer is obvious:

QUITTING ISN'T ABOUT WILLPOWER

How do you react when people tell you that you have to change your ways and sort out your drinking problem? Don't you find you tend to do the opposite? Wouldn't you describe that as wilful? In fact, it tends to be the most strong-willed people who find it hardest to quit by using the willpower method, because when the door fails to open they won't give up and they'll force themselves to keep pushing on the hinges until they can push no more.

IN HER OWN WORDS: JENNY

I managed to go 18 months without drinking. I knew it would be hard at the beginning, but I was determined to get through those first few weeks and then I was sure it would get easier. Looking back, the first weeks weren't the hardest. I was so determined and I did everything I could to avoid alcohol. Pretty soon I'd gone six weeks without touching a drop. But I could feel my resolve weakening. I had made the effort to avoid the booze aisle in the supermarket and steer clear of bars, but there's only so long you can keep that up. Normal life takes over and inevitably you find yourself faced with temptation.

Christmas came at a good time. It gave me a new target and I was able to strengthen my resolve. I made it through still dry, despite finding myself in several situations where alcohol was flowing freely. But it wasn't getting any easier; it was getting harder. With each milestone I passed, the end of the road seemed further away. I began to doubt my ability to keep it up.

The approach of my second Christmas finished me off. I was cooking one afternoon when I found a bottle of vodka in a cupboard that I'd forgotten about. I wept as I poured myself a glass and I trembled as I put it to my lips. I was overwhelmed by a sense of failure and I collapsed in floods of tears. Not only had I endured 18 months of hardship for nothing, I was now convinced that I would be a slave to alcohol for the rest of my life.

After I quit with Easyway I was able to understand that the end of the road seemed to be getting further away because, in fact, there was no end to the road. With the willpower method there is no moment of escape—it's a lifetime's struggle.

GETTING THERE THE EASY WAY

With Easyway, you arrive at your goal as soon as you remove the desire to drink and stop drinking. You remove the desire by understanding that alcohol does nothing for you whatsoever and that there is nothing to fear about life as a nondrinker. By now you should be quite clear on both these points. If you continue to believe that you are making a sacrifice, you will never reach the end of the road.

The willpower method doesn't only make it harder to quit, it actually encourages you to stay hooked because:

1. It reinforces the myth that quitting is hard and, therefore, adds to your fear.

2. It creates a feeling of deprivation, which you will seek to alleviate in your usual way—by drinking. It makes alcohol seem even more precious.

Failing to quit using the willpower method makes it harder to try again because, like Jenny, you will have reinforced the belief that it is impossible to cure your problem. Jenny wept bitter tears when she first gave in and had that drink of vodka.

Other people who fail with the willpower method say they felt an enormous sense of relief when they had that first drink but that it didn't make them happy. In fact, it made them even more miserable. Anyone who tells you it's a pleasure is confusing pleasure with the relief of ending their pain. No one thinks, "Great! I've fallen back into the alcohol trap." It is not a pleasure; it is a deeply upsetting experience, full of guilt, shame, fear, and hopelessness.

OTHER QUITTERS

The testimony of other quitters who use the willpower method can be damaging to your own desire to quit. They break down into two types: the Braggers and the Whiners. They either brag about the sacrifices they're making or they whine about them. Either way, they reinforce the myth that quitting demands sacrifice.

FIFTH INSTRUCTION: IGNORE ANY ADVICE THAT CONFLICTS WITH EASYWAY

That includes the advice of anyone who claims to have quit by the willpower method. Contrary to what they may tell you, there is no sacrifice. You are making great progress toward becoming a nondrinker without any need for willpower. All you have had to do is follow a simple set of instructions. It should now be clear in your mind that you are not "giving up" anything. Alcohol does nothing for you whatsoever. Drinkers only think it does because addiction creates the illusion of pleasure. That "pleasure" is nothing more than the partial and temporary relief from the craving, which was caused by the drug in the first place.

When you understand the way addiction works, you lose the fear of success. Take away the fear and you win the tug of war. It's easy.

Jenny was waiting for the moment when the hardship ended and she became a happy, relaxed nondrinker. But with Easyway there is nothing to wait for. You become a happy nondrinker the moment you remove the desire to drink.

The third instruction was to begin your attempt to quit with a feeling of elation. This is the most important decision of your life. By quitting you are choosing a life of health and happiness over one of sickness and misery. If you've followed all the instructions and understood everything you've read so far, you should be feeling a sense of elation and eagerness to finish the job. You've taken a major step in freeing yourself from slavery to alcohol. You can start living your life again, in control and free.

If you still have doubts, then you have either missed something, in which case you need to go back and reread anything you are stuck on, or there is one last piece of brainwashing that is preventing you from feeling the sense of elation.

Some people who try and fail to stop with the willpower method don't conclude that they are weak-willed but that their failure must be down to another aspect of their personality over which they have no control. When all other explanations fail them, there is one theory that conveniently provides the excuse they need to stay in the trap: the so-called "addictive personality" theory.

SUMMARY

- **People who try to quit with the willpower method never win the tug of war. They always believe they're being deprived**

- **Addiction is not a symptom of being weak-willed. In fact, it is often the opposite**

- **With the willpower method, you never reach your goal**

- **People who brag or whine about quitting with willpower still believe they are making a sacrifice**

- **With Easyway, you reach your goal the moment you reverse the brainwashing and stop drinking**

- **You are not "giving up" anything**

- **FIFTH INSTRUCTION: IGNORE ANY ADVICE THAT CONFLICTS WITH EASYWAY**

Chapter 10

I HAVE AN ADDICTIVE PERSONALITY

The character traits shared by addicts are not the cause of their addiction; they are the result of it.

Scientists always seem to be searching for proof that our behavior is beyond our control. Despite compelling evidence that events that occur in our early years have a strong influence on the way we behave as adults, there is a determination to find a genetic link to everything from happiness to homicide. You don't need a scientist to tell you that both nature and nurture play a part in who we turn out to be and how we behave—that's abundantly clear. It's also proven that our behavioral tendencies can be altered at any stage in life. In short, your personality was not fixed at birth.

The addictive personality theory, or the belief that a genetic predisposition to addiction plays a part, is a godsend for hopeless addicts who refuse to open their minds to the possibility that there is an easy cure. All the other excuses we make so that we can keep drinking are lame and we know it—we feel pathetic hearing ourselves say them—but the addictive personality or genetic predisposition excuse is different. It has science behind it! We can say it with gravitas and truly believe what we're saying.

The thinking goes like this: Some people have a flaw in their genetic make-up that makes them more susceptible than most to becoming addicted. This gives us an excuse to avoid our fear of success by not even trying to quit and it allows us to pity ourselves rather than despise ourselves, as we continue to slide deeper and deeper into the trap.

THE ADDICTIVE PERSONALITY THEORY DOESN'T SOLVE YOUR PROBLEM; IT MERELY CEMENTS IT AND JUSTIFIES IT

Do you want to believe that you were born with a genetic predisposition to self-destruction? Did you believe that before you started drinking? The fact that you picked up this book suggests you believe you can be cured. So where does that leave the addictive personality theory or the belief that some kind of genetic predisposition to addiction plays an important part in your imprisonment?

A few so-called experts have bandied the term "addictive personality" about so often that it's easy to be fooled into believing it's an established condition. It is not. It's a theory and nothing more, largely based on the number of people who have multiple addictions, e.g. drinkers who are also smokers or gamblers, or heroin addicts who smoke and are heavily in debt.

Smoking, drinking, gambling, overeating, debt—they do seem to coincide in a lot of people, don't they? In the next chapter we will look at how people try to cure one addiction by substituting it with another and why that is doomed to failure. For now, please get it clear in your mind: All these addictions *are* caused by the same thing, but it's nothing to do with your personality or genes. It's the misguided belief that the thing you are addicted to gives you a genuine pleasure or crutch.

BIG MONSTER OR PERSONALITY?

Addiction is a lonely condition, despite the fact that it affects millions of people. Addicts become very insular and convince themselves that they are suffering with a problem that's unique to them. That's why talking to other addicts is so beneficial: It makes you realize that they are experiencing, or have experienced, exactly what you are going through, and you begin to see that addiction is not a weakness in the individual but a weakness in the society that brainwashes individuals into the trap.

Just like the belief that you lack the willpower to quit, the addictive personality theory or belief that a genetic predisposition to addiction might keep you trapped is reinforced by failed attempts. If you put all your effort into something but still fail, it's natural to assume that it's beyond your power to solve. Similarly, the Braggers and Whiners who claim to have quit by the willpower method also add weight to the theory. They can go months or even years without a drink yet still crave it! That can't be the effect of alcohol in their system—it must be their personality, right?

Wrong. They didn't crave alcohol before they started drinking. The craving has nothing to do with their personality; it is the Big Monster, which they have failed to destroy.

Remember, the Little Monster is the restless feeling you get when you're withdrawing from alcohol; the Big Monster is triggered by that and asserts that drinking gives some sort of pleasure or crutch and the only way to relieve the restless feeling is to consume more alcohol. When you have another drink, the discomfort appears to temporarily disappear, and so the Big Monster is strengthened. The willpower method focuses only on killing the Little Monster. It ignores the Big Monster and, in fact, makes it stronger by encouraging the belief that you are making a sacrifice.

It's not only the Little Monster that can arouse the Big Monster; all sorts of things can create a restless feeling that triggers it: a trauma, a social occasion, hunger, a smell, a picture... as long as you allow the Big Monster to remain alive in your head, you will always be vulnerable to a feeling of deprivation and a craving for forbidden fruit. Braggers and Whiners kill off the Little Monster within days of quitting, but they never kill the Big Monster.

Killing the Big Monster is easy provided you keep an open mind. If you cling to the excuse that you have an addictive personality or that some kind of genetic predisposition prevents your escape, it means that your mind is not open and you risk sentencing yourself to a lifetime of slavery. The simple truth is that whatever your personality or genetics, you will find it easy to stop, and stay stopped, as long as you use THE RIGHT METHOD: EASYWAY.

FILLING A VOID

If addiction is nothing to do with personality, why do some people fall deeper into the trap than others? Why can one person have the occasional drink while another downs the whole bottle and opens another? Doesn't that suggest that one has a personality that's more prone to addiction than the other?

It does point to a difference between them, yes, but the difference lies in their conditioning, not in their genetic make-up. We are conditioned by all sorts of things: parental guidance, peer pressure, education, income, opportunity… in Chapter Three we explained about the void—a sense of emptiness and insecurity which opens up at birth and that we spend our lives trying to fill. For some people the void is greater than for others because of their upbringing, the environment in which they live, and a whole host of other factors. Such factors might determine how easily they are drawn to drink and then how much and how often they drink.

The restrictions in our lives also control our drinking. Some people only drink one unit a week because that's all they can afford. Some have time to drink in their lunch break, others don't. But if all the restrictions were taken out of our way, we would all tend toward drinking more, not less, because that's how addiction works.

Look at the people who fall deepest into the trap and you'll find they are the ones with the greatest opportunity, the most money, and the greatest desire because of the way they have been conditioned. You may regard them as hopeless cases. Easyway has seen countless such "hopeless cases" released from the trap simply by reversing the conditioning, unraveling the brainwashing, and helping them to realize that their little crutch is actually no such thing—it is their mortal enemy.

You may also have noticed that people who don't fall into the trap at all—those lucky ones who can happily say no to a drink—seem to be a different breed. They make you feel slightly uncomfortable, don't they? You feel much more at home with your fellow addicts and you appear to share similar character traits. You might take this to mean that there's a shared personality trait that has led to you all having a drink problem. But what are those traits? An unstable temperament, which swings between exuberance and misery, a tendency toward excess, a high susceptibility to stress, evasiveness, anxiety, insecurity? These traits are all caused by drinking; they are not the reason you drink.

THE DESIRE FOR ALCOHOL IS CAUSED
BY DRINKING ALCOHOL

People with a drink problem feel more comfortable in the company of other drinkers for one simple reason: They won't challenge you or make you think twice about your addiction because they're in the same boat. All addicts know that they're doing something stupid and self-destructive. If you're surrounded by other people doing the same thing, you don't feel quite so foolish.

One of the best things about getting free from alcohol addiction is that you also get free from the harmful effect it has on your character. You'll be able to enjoy the company of all sorts of people, drinkers and nondrinkers, and you'll realize that non-drinkers stay interesting for longer.

You just need to understand that you didn't become addicted to alcohol because you have an addictive personality. If you think you have an addictive personality, it's simply because you got addicted to alcohol. This is the trick that addiction plays on you. It makes you feel that you're dependent on alcohol and that there's some weakness in your character or genetic make-up. It distorts your perceptions and thus maintains its grip on you.

DEFYING LOGIC

Let's say there was a gene that predisposed people to become addicts. It would be safe to assume that this gene would have appeared in a fairly constant percentage of the world population and in the same geographical concentrations throughout history, would it not? Yet this is not the case. Smoking statistics, for example, paint a very different picture: In the U.S.A., adult smoking peaked in 1954 at 45 percent, but it was down to 14 percent by 2017. A similar trend is seen to be evident throughout most of western

Europe. As regards women smokers, there were only a handful of them, for example, in the U.S.A.—it had been a political gesture to smoke for suffragettes —before Lucky Strike started to aim advertising at women, with ads featuring the likes of Amelia Earhart in the 1920s always emphasizing the "slimming effects"—another myth!—of smoking. By 1965, it was 39 percent of women who smoked as the first cigarette aimed exclusively at women came along, namely, Virginia Slims (slogan: "You've come a long way, baby"). Currently the number of women smokers in western Europe stands at around 22 percent. In the U.S.A., in 2017, the figure was 12.2 percent.

So are we to conclude that the proportion of people with addictive personalities has changed massively in just a few decades?

At the same time, the number of smokers in Asia has soared. What complex genetic anomaly is this that rises and falls so rapidly, and even appears to transfer itself wholesale from one continent to another?

Even if you did have a genetic predisposition to addiction, it simply doesn't mean that escape is impossible or even more difficult for you. Nor does it mean that you're more likely to fall back into the trap. The great news about addiction is that it's easy to break free WHEN YOU KNOW HOW.

KNOW YOUR ENEMY

You are engaged in a battle against two monsters. Your chances of winning that battle will be greatly improved if you get to know those monsters inside out. Understand how they work and what they want, and you will find it easy to conquer them.

The Little Monster was created the first time you drank alcohol. It feeds on alcohol and when you don't give it what it wants, it begins to complain. This feeling is barely perceptible, like a slight itch, but it is enough to arouse the Big Monster.

This Big Monster is not physical but psychological. It is created by all the brainwashing that has led you to believe that alcohol gives you pleasure or a crutch and it interprets the Little Monster's complaints as "I need a drink." Trying to please the Big Monster means trying to satisfy a craving by doing the very thing that caused the craving in the first place.

Every time you have a drink it temporarily quietens the Little Monster, creating the illusion that the alcohol has made you relaxed and happy. In fact, all it has done is taken you from feeling miserable and restless to feeling OK. Now you will need it again and again just to keep you feeling OK. But actually you never quite get back to where you were before you started. Look again at the diagram in Chapter 4. Every time you give your body a poison, it develops a tolerance against it. So every time you consume alcohol you need to consume more to get the same boost, and every time you stop you sink lower. The longer you go on trying to satisfy the Little Monster with alcohol, the lower you sink and the more dependent you feel.

While the Little Monster is barely perceptible, the Big Monster really can make you miserable. When it is awakened, it fills your head with thoughts that trigger the very physical sensation of deprivation. You only get that feeling of deprivation if you feel that you're missing out on something.

EMBRACE THE TRUTH

Your drink problem has nothing to do with your personality and everything to do with the brainwashing you've been subjected to from birth. The craving is nothing more than a desire to feel the way a nondrinker feels all the time, but the thought of "giving up" drink is frightening if you believe that it gives you pleasure or a crutch. This conflict leaves you feeling helpless and confused. You wish you could just take control of the situation and sort yourself out.

The hopelessness of the prison makes addicts try to blot out the problem and pretend it doesn't exist. They lie to themselves about the state they're in and laugh it off with other addicts, but deep down you know it's no laughing matter. It's a miserable situation and if you could end it with a wave of a magic wand, you would not hesitate. So hiding behind the theory of the addictive personality and genetics is futile. You might be able to fool other people, but you can't fool yourself.

Using any excuse just so you can continue drinking means consigning yourself to a lifetime of slavery and the risk of serious health problems. Release yourself from the prison. Take your head out of the sand and see things as they really are. There is a wonderful life awaiting you, free from alcohol. You don't need a magic wand; you have something in your hands that's just as effective when it comes to curing addiction: Easyway. All you have to do is follow the instructions.

1. Follow all the instructions

2. Keep an open mind

3. Begin with a feeling of elation

4. Never doubt your decision to quit

5. Ignore any advice that conflicts with Easyway

If you've followed all the instructions in order, then you've already taken a big step towards freedom. You have overcome denial and accepted that you have an addiction to alcohol. You have also taken action to do something about the problem. That's another big step. Now all you have to do is kill the Big Monster. Once the Big Monster is dead, you will find it easy to cut off the supply to the Little Monster and it will die very quickly. Remember, people who try to quit with the willpower method never kill the Big Monster; they think it's enough just to kill the Little Monster.

You've already begun to kill the Big Monster and you understand that the way to finish it off is by understanding the way the alcohol trap works. We are brainwashed by parents, friends, role models, the alcoholic drinks industry, the medical profession, governments, and other so-called experts, all of whom were themselves brainwashed by other influences of their own. Some of us are brainwashed more than others, but all alcohol addicts are in the same trap and there is only one way out, which is the same for everybody:

UNDO THE BRAINWASHING AND STOP DRINKING ALCOHOL!

At this stage a lot of people say they understand everything we've said completely and are in a hurry to get to the end, but it often turns out that they still retain some belief in the illusion of pleasure or crutch. As long as you believe the illusion you will always be susceptible to feeling deprived. It's essential, therefore, that we make sure you remove all the illusions completely and start trusting your instincts.

SUMMARY

- **The addictive personality is a myth that gives the addict an excuse to avoid even trying to escape**

- **Personality and genetics really don't matter**

- **The personality traits shared by addicts are caused by their addiction; they are not the cause**

- **Once you accept that there is a cure for your drink problem, then you can set about getting free**

- **In order to get free forever, you have to kill the Big Monster**

Chapter 11

SUBSTITUTES

IN THIS CHAPTER
•*THE SUBSTITUTE THEORY* •*FLAWED LOGIC* •*CUTTING DOWN*
•*BREAK THE CHAIN*

Perhaps you think you can solve your problem by finding an alternative to alcohol. This won't cure your addiction. In fact, it will force you deeper into the trap.

The willpower method is based on the theory that if you can resist the temptation to drink for long enough, your body will readjust to not having alcohol and the craving will stop. It assumes that the hardest thing about quitting is the physical withdrawal as you purge your body of the drug.

It only takes a few days to purge your body of alcohol, yet anyone who has tried to stop drinking with the willpower method will know that the craving goes on much longer than that and even intensifies. That's because you never tackle the mental aspect that accounts for 99 percent of addiction—you never kill the Big Monster.

Nevertheless, the willpower method continues to be prescribed by doctors and other so-called experts and to help you tackle the withdrawal they recommend substitutes. With other drugs like nicotine and heroin, they encourage addicts to take the drug in a different, "cleaner" form; for example, nicotine patches or gum or more recently e-cigarettes. The theory is that you can keep getting the drug without the harmful smoke while you concentrate on breaking the "habit" and then, when you're ready, you can gradually cut down the dose of nicotine until you're able to get by without it altogether.

They call this nicotine replacement therapy (NRT) and it sounds straightforward, doesn't it? But NRT has been an abject failure. Just like the e-cigarettes and other alternatives peddled for vast sums by the tobacco industry, the NRT solutions recommended by the medical profession only keep smokers hooked on nicotine.

The great irony of NRT solutions is that they actually enable smokers to get nicotine at times when they would otherwise make do without it, such as on flights and in restaurants. Far from being the key to their prison, NRT keeps them more firmly locked in.

In the case of alcohol, the so-called experts haven't yet come up with an alternative form of administering the drug without the harmful side effects, but drinkers who try to quit with the willpower method will often replace alcohol with other drugs, most commonly nicotine or refined sugar. We refer to sugar as a drug because it has

> *"Because alcohol is encouraged by our culture, we get the idea that it isn't dangerous. However, alcohol is the most potent and most toxic of the legal psychoactive drugs... Alcohol is a make-you-stupid drug."*
>
> **Beverly A. Potter and Sebastian Orfali,** *Brain Boosters*

very much the same addictive effect as other drugs.

When drinkers feel the craving for alcohol, they smoke a cigarette or eat a piece of candy instead. Sooner or later, they believe, they will break their drinking "habit," then they can come off the cigarettes or candy and they'll be cured.

> • Larger wine glasses encourage more drinking. For many years, a standard U.S. wine glass was eight ounces and you were supposed to fill it with a five-ounce serving of wine (equal to 127 calories per glass of red, incidentally). In recent years, 12- to 16-ounce glasses have become the norm, not only in restaurants and bars, but also in many private residences.
>
> • Drinkers have a tendency to overpour white wine (rather than red), perhaps because it's less "visible" in the glass. People also tend to pour more wine into glasses they're holding in their hands than into glasses on the tabletop.

FLAWED LOGIC

There are three fatal flaws in this approach that explain why the substitute theory fails:

1. Problem drinking is not a habit; it's an addiction.

2. The physical effects of withdrawal are negligible. Addiction is 99 percent mental.

3. Substituting alcohol with nicotine or sugar is just swapping one addiction for another.

Drinkers, like smokers, think the ritual they go through is part of the enjoyment they get from drinking. Opening the bottle, choosing a glass, pouring the drink, sniffing it, holding it up to the light, swirling it around, swilling it in their mouth... the way they hold the glass, the way they place it down, the way they bring it to their lips... these are the ritualistic tics that make drinkers think they're doing more than mere drug taking. The truth is the only reason they go through the ritual is to get the alcohol and the belief that it gives them some sort of pleasure or crutch is purely the Big Monster playing tricks on them.

Let's go back to the heroin addict. Most people hate injections. But the heroin addict can't wait for that moment when the needle pierces her skin. Is that because she's anticipating a tremendous high? Or is it because she knows it will end the terrible panic and misery she's suffering, if only for a short time?

Heroin addicts are under no

> *"Like a lot of moms at the end of a long day, I turned to the internet and my nightly wine... I somehow didn't see it when my one glass of wine turned into five each night. The normalization of mommy wino culture memes and the parade of articles on mom sites shouting out the benefits of drinking helped justify my own growing problem."*
> **Sarah Cottrell, babble**

illusion that they enjoy injecting themselves. The only pleasure they get from it is the relief of knowing they are getting their fix of the drug and they do it as fast as they can. Similarly, there is no ritualistic pleasure in taking off tight shoes. You pull them off as soon as you get the chance in order to relieve the pain.

When you regard alcohol as a pleasure or crutch, you feel deprived if you can't have it. The willpower method is designed to make you overcome this feeling of deprivation. In reality, it intensifies it. Taking a substitute when you feel the craving for alcohol may momentarily take away the feeling of deprivation, but it doesn't remove the illusion of alcohol being a pleasure or crutch. As long as that belief remains in your mind, any little trigger can arouse it. The fact is, within moments of using the substitute the craving begins again. This time it's twofold... one is the alcohol, the other the craving for the addictive substitute the addict is attempting to use.

Substitutes just keep the Big Monster alive.

It's actually very easy to overcome the physical pangs of withdrawal. These are the cries of the Little Monster and they are barely perceptible. You already know what the physical withdrawal feels like because you experience it every time you have a drink. It's a faint, restless feeling, like mild hunger. If your mind is occupied with something else, you don't even notice it. The problem arises when those faint cries arouse the Big Monster in your mind. Now you can't concentrate on anything else until you've satisfied the craving. As long as you resist the desire, you will feel deprived and miserable, like a child throwing a tantrum.

So you appease the child with a piece of candy. Now you no longer feel deprived, but you haven't satisfied the Little Monster and soon the Big Monster is grumbling again. So you have another candy and another and another. Before you know it, you have an eating problem to add to your drink problem.

CUTTING DOWN

Let's imagine that you reach a point where you think you have broken the "habit" and you're ready to reduce the dose of the drug. As a purely physical process, this is doomed to fail. When you understand how addiction works, you know that the tendency is always to crave more, not less, because of the tolerance you build up in defense against the poison. The more tolerance you build up, the bigger the dose you need to get the relief you're craving. By gradually reducing your intake, you don't get near the relief you crave, so your desire increases and you actually make quitting harder. It makes the drug more precious, not less.

Killing the Little Monster is easy: Simply deny it its fix completely and it will die very quickly. You don't have to give it all your concentration or apply any willpower. When you feel those faint cries, instead of interpreting them as "I need a drink," just picture the Little Monster squirming and dying inside you and enjoy the feeling for what it is—the Little Monster starving to death.

Killing the Little Monster is only hard if you fail to destroy the Big Monster. It is the Big Monster that interprets those tiny cries as "I need a drink" and causes you to feel deprived and miserable if you can't have one.

> *"Until about ten years ago, my patients with alcoholic liver disease were mostly middle-aged men. But women now make up about half of my caseload. It used to be that patients were in their forties and fifties when I first saw them. But I'm now seeing sizeable and rising numbers of women in their twenties. Some have irreversible liver damage. [Then there are]... the steady drinkers. Typically they have a half-bottle of wine with their meal every night, or at lunchtime, and another drink at dinner. They are never drunk, but they drink in a sustained manner. They don't realize they have a problem because they think alcoholics are down-and-outs, or pub regulars. They have wine with their meal and because of that they somehow think that takes away the harm, or they say, 'But I don't drink spirits.'"*
>
> Dr. Gray Smith-Laing,
> Medway Maritime Hospital, Kent, England

It's not the "habit" of drinking that you need to break before you kill the Little Monster; it's the desire. You remove the desire by recognizing that any sense of alcohol giving you pleasure or a crutch is an illusion brought on by brainwashing and that the only thing standing between you and genuine pleasure is your next drink. If you fail to remove the desire for alcohol, you can will yourself to abstain for long enough to kill the Little Monster, but other triggers such as hunger or stress will stir the Big Monster into making you think, "I need a drink."

For the addict who thinks she's broken the "habit" of drinking by pacifying the craving with other drugs, this is devastating. You think you've overcome the physical withdrawal, but suddenly there you are craving your fix again. This is only a problem if you don't understand the nature of the trap you are in. With Easyway, you remove the desire completely before you kill the Little Monster.

BREAK THE CHAIN

The main reason why any drinker wants to quit is to get free from the slavery of alcohol addiction. That is the thing that makes drinkers miserable when they fail to quit—a feeling of frustration and helplessness, like being chained up without any hope of escape. There are many other depressing aspects to drinking: the ill health, the waste of money, the embarrassing behavior, to name but three; but when you find yourself reaching for that bottle despite promising yourself you wouldn't, or pouring another glass even though you swore you'd just have the one—what drinker wouldn't want to rid herself of that misery?

BY USING SUBSTITUTES YOU CONSIGN YOURSELF TO A LIFETIME OF SLAVERY

One of the arguments the medical profession uses to promote nicotine substitutes is that, even if they don't break your nicotine addiction, at least they don't fill you with all the other harmful poisons associated with smoking. In other words, their method for getting you off one set of poisons is to keep you hooked on another.

Any substitute you use to replace alcohol may spare you

the hangovers, aching liver, incontinence, and other unpleasant side-effects, but it will bring its own new set of problems. Choose cigarettes to try to satisfy your alcohol cravings and you will quickly get hooked on a drug that is the world's biggest killer and will cost you a fortune. Choose candy and you're buying into a substance that is responsible for a global obesity and diabetes epidemic. You multiply your problems. Substitutes simply don't work.

THE GREAT EVIL OF ALL SUBSTITUTES, WHATEVER THEY MAY BE, IS THAT THEY PERPETUATE THE ILLUSION THAT YOU'RE MAKING A SACRIFICE WHEN YOU QUIT

It's essential that you remove this illusion and to help you with that, let's look more closely at the people who do most to promote it: so-called normal drinkers.

SUMMARY

- **Your alcohol problem is not a habit; it's an addiction**
- **Addiction is 1 percent physical and 99 percent mental**
- **Substitutes perpetuate the illusion that you're making a sacrifice when you quit**
- **You don't need substitutes when you have no desire to drink**

Chapter 12

NORMAL DRINKERS

We have established that, like all drinkers, you want to feel the way a nondrinker feels all the time. It's pointless then to envy any other drinker.

Say you have a tile missing from your roof and rain is dripping in and threatening to ruin the carpets. All you have to do is have the tile replaced and the problem is solved, immediately and permanently. It might take a little time to clear up the mess, but you will find the clear-up process much easier knowing that the leak has been repaired.

You can cure a drink problem just as easily by stopping the flow of alcohol. As soon as you do, you know your problem is solved and you can enjoy the process of repairing the damage.

But say you don't replace the roof tile and choose instead just to put buckets under the leak. You might slow down the rate of damage to the inside of your house, but you have the constant headache of having to empty buckets and replace them. How long are you prepared to keep doing this? Do you expect the hole in the roof to just fix itself one day?

Of course, it won't. In fact, sooner or later another tile is blown away and the hole doubles in size. Now you're struggling to catch all the drips and your buckets are overflowing before you can empty them.

As time goes on the flow of water gets heavier and heavier, and the damage to your house is becoming disastrous. But you can make it stop any time you want simply by fixing the roof.

Now, would it make any sense for a person with two tiles missing to think, "I wish I only had one tile missing?" Surely they'd be better off fixing the roof properly! That describes exactly the situation if you make the mistake of envying "normal drinkers."

Advertisers use glamor to sell alcohol, but the truth is quite different. Here are some of the main effects of alcohol on your looks:

• Makes your face puffy

• Weight gain and tired eyes

• Accelerates your skin's natural ageing process—parches your system, including the skin. It dries your skin from within, leading to wrinkles

- Enlarges the blood vessels on your face, adding red blotches

- Dehydrates your hair, giving it a straw-like quality

We all know people who seem to be able to enjoy a drink whenever they want without getting out of control. Problem drinkers envy these so-called normal drinkers and wish they could pick and choose when and how much they drank in the same way. Rather than recognizing drinking as a source of misery that does nothing for them whatsoever, they still believe it gives them some sort of pleasure or crutch and find the idea of quitting completely quite disturbing.

We often find ourselves having this conversation with women who come to Easyway looking for a cure for drinking. They begin by asking us, "Do you ever desire a drink?"

"Never," we say.

"Do you think you could have an occasional drink and not get hooked again?" they ask.

"I could, but what would be the point, since I have no desire to drink alcohol?"

"Could you teach me to have an occasional drink without getting hooked again?"

"Sure. I could teach you the same trick with arsenic if you like."

"Why on Earth would I want to do that?"

"Exactly."

It's wonderful to see the look on their face as they make the connection. They've begun the conversation with the belief that alcohol provides some benefit and we've ended it by opening their eyes to the fact that alcohol is nothing but poison. When the client realizes this, the fear they have about never drinking again —the fear of success—disappears. Just by seeing the facts in a new light, they go from fear to joy in an instant.

FEAR: "I will never be able to drink again."

JOY: "I never have to drink again."

Actually, we've been unfair. Alcohol is not just a poison. For the sake of balance we should point out that it does have three genuine uses:

- as an antiseptic

- as a detergent

- as a fuel

Similar to denatured alcohol, in fact. Would you drink meths and believe it was doing you good? The one thing you don't want to do with alcohol is take it internally because:

- It's a powerful poison—half a pint drunk neat will kill you

- It's a diuretic—a drink that makes you thirsty

- It's a highly addictive drug—90 percent of adults are hooked

- It's a drain on your finances—an average drinker spends more than $90,000 on booze in a lifetime

- It impedes judgment and concentration

- It weakens your immune system

- It destroys your nervous system

- It causes stress

- It tastes foul

So why do we envy those "normal" drinkers who haven't suffered the effects of alcohol like we have? Well, for that very reason alone, you might say. But then, why not envy a nondrinker? They haven't had their life ruined by alcohol either. If you think it's better to be a "normal" drinker than a nondrinker, you must still believe there is some benefit to drinking.

Drinkers who try to cut down know that there's danger in drinking, but they think they can limit the threat by limiting the amount they drink.

Rather than flying free, they create a number of serious problems for themselves:

1. They keep themselves addicted to alcohol.

2. They wish their lives away waiting for the next drink.

3. Instead of relieving the withdrawal pangs whenever they feel like it, they force themselves to endure the discomfort and so are permanently restless.

4. They reinforce the illusion that drinking is enjoyable.

THE ILLUSION OF CONTROL?

"Normal" drinkers give the impression of being in control. That's the difference between them and you: While drinking controls you, they seem to be able to decide when they drink and how much without any trouble at all. But is that really the case? Remember, all drinkers lie in order to give the impression that they are in control.

The fly on the upper slope of the pitcher plant thinks it's in control. It knows it can fly away at any moment. But it doesn't. It continues to drink, sliding further and further into the plant, until it's too late. Anyone observing this will know that the fly is doomed the moment it lands on the lip of the plant. If it was really in control, it would have flown away. But the fly is controlled by the pitcher plant from the moment it picks up the scent of the nectar.

To the heavy drinker, all "normal" drinkers appear to be in control. But would you say a pilot was in control if he was flying through a mountain range with inaccurate charts and his instruments had been tampered with? He might have his hands on the controls but each decision he made would be based on false information. He would be unaware of the danger and so would have no fear, but that doesn't mean the danger didn't exist.

In the Hitchcock movie *Notorious*, the heroine is being nursed through illness by her husband. Or she thinks she is. Then she discovers that she's not really ill; he's poisoning her. She tries to escape, but the drug is taking away the use of her legs and leaving her mind addled. Sound familiar? The husband is using some poison other than alcohol, but the similarity is stark.

While the wife thinks she's being nursed by her husband, she has no fear of the food he's giving her. She thinks it's doing her good. "Normal" drinkers have no fear of alcohol for the same reason. They think it's giving them pleasure. Like the heroine and like the fly on the upper slope of the pitcher plant, they are oblivious to the danger they're in. By the time they realize they are in a trap, they are way beyond the point where they lost control.

If this sounds extreme, it's supposed to. The effects of alcohol can be every bit as catastrophic as the poison for the wife and the pitcher plant for the fly, but there is one crucial difference: The person administering the poison is you. You have the power to stop any time you choose.

RASH DECISIONS

Imagine you have a spot on your face. Someone lends you an ointment that they say will clear it up, so you rub it on and sure enough the spot disappears. A week later, the spot's back and it's bigger and redder this time. You apply more ointment and it disappears again. Five days later, the spot returns, but now it's more than just a spot, it's a rash. You apply more ointment, but as time goes on the rash returns sooner and sooner and it's bigger and itchier each time. Imagine how desperate you'd feel knowing that it's going to get worse and worse until you can find a cure. You're also so reliant on that jar of ointment that you're prepared to pay a fortune for it and you're afraid to go anywhere without it.

You then read an article in your newspaper and discover this is not only happening to you: Thousands of other people are using this ointment and it has been proved that, far from curing the problem, it is the ointment that is causing it to grow. All the ointment does is to take the initial spot beneath the skin, at which point the spot feeds on the ointment and returns to the surface with a vengeance. All you have to do to get rid of the spot is to stop using the ointment. Do that and the spot will disappear of its own accord in a few days.

How would you feel? Would you feel miserable that you could never use the ointment again, or would you be elated that you never had to? Do you think you'd need to use any willpower to stop using the ointment? Of course not!

Can you see how this scenario applies to alcohol?

Everyone who uses alcohol does so in the false belief that it is helping them in some way. The only way to stop feeling a need for alcohol is to stop using it. See alcohol as clearly as you see that ointment. Rejoice in the fact that you are on the verge of being set free from the whole filthy nightmare.

THE CATAPULT

When you pull a rubber band, it stretches easily at first but gets more resistant the more you stretch it. The same effect takes place when you try to control your drinking.

You are now very familiar with the two monsters and how they influence your drinking. When you try to control your alcohol intake, you resist the cries of the Little Monster a little longer than normal. What effect do you think that has on your desire for alcohol? Just as the pull in the elastic band increases the more you stretch it,

THE LONGER YOU RESIST THE DESIRE FOR SOMETHING, THE GREATER THE DESIRE BECOMES

The more you deny yourself a drink, the more deprived you'll feel and the more miserable you'll become. You find it easy at first when you're fired up with determination to cut down, but it gets harder and harder the longer you go on. You won't give in to this hardship, though, because another part of your brain is feeling rather pleased with itself for taking control of the situation. This creates a contradictory dialogue in your mind. One part of your brain is whining about not being able to drink; another is keeping a haughty superiority as it controls the rations. The result is a constant gabble, dominating your mind with thoughts of your next drink.

BEING DOMINATED BY ALCOHOL AND BEING IN CONTROL OF IT ARE DIRECT OPPOSITES

Now another force comes into effect. Because you are reducing the dose of poison and the money you waste on booze, the ill-effects are waning and your antipathy towards drinking is reduced. On the one hand your desire for alcohol is increasing; on the other you're starting to forget your reasons for cutting down. Both lead to the same inevitable outcome: a return to drinking. The elastic pings back and catapults you deeper into the trap than you were before.

DRINKERS WHO TRY TO CONTROL THEIR DRINKING TEND TO END UP DRINKING MORE

BEHIND THE MASK

You don't have to look very hard to see through the veneer of pleasure and control worn by "normal" drinkers. For example, watch their behavior when the question arises of who's going to drive. On the face of it they discuss the issue with casual indifference.

"Am I driving tonight, darling?"

"I will if you want. I don't mind."

"Really? Are you sure it's not my turn?"

"I can't remember. I don't mind, honestly. I'll drive, you enjoy yourself."

"Well, if you insist. I think I will."

But we know what they're really thinking, don't we? The opening question, "Am I driving tonight, darling?" is cleverly designed to elicit the answer "no." But the partner doesn't come back with a straightforward "no," he throws the responsibility back on her: "I will if you want." Then he adds, "I don't mind," meaning, "It's a big disappointment, but I'll stomach it."

She expresses her relief by faking surprise at his gallantry. "Really?" Then, graciously offers him the chance to change his mind: "Are you sure it's not my turn?" Of course, for him to say, "Yes, it is your turn," would be extremely ungallant, so he feigns ignorance: "I can't remember." Then he repeats the plaintive "I don't mind," hoping she'll take pity on him and feel guilty, and rubs it in with "you enjoy yourself," implying that there's no chance of enjoying oneself without drinking. She reaffirms this with, "I think I will," and the first thing she does is top up her glass. She can't wait to relieve her craving.

Both partners are like prisoners drawing lots for the gallows. Neither wants to come across as so desperate to drink that they'll say, "You drive, I really have to drink tonight," yet the relief of the one and the despondency of the other when it's all resolved is plain to see.

The "normal" drinker claims to get pleasure from drinking, but ask them to define that pleasure and all they offer you is defensive excuses:

"I can take it or leave it."

"I don't drink that much."

"It's not doing me any harm."

If you genuinely enjoy a drink, why would you choose to leave it? If drinking is a genuine pleasure, why wait so long in between? The only possible reason is that you fear the effects of drinking— in which case, why do it at all?

FEAR AND PLEASURE DO NOT GO HAND IN HAND

It's an annual tradition among many "normal" drinkers to abstain from drinking throughout January, ostensibly to "detox" after the heavy drinking of Christmas. There's a recent trend to do the same at other times of the year also. What are these abstainers trying to prove? That drink isn't a problem for them. What are they actually proving? That it is.

If they didn't think drink was a problem, why go without for a whole month? Imagine if a friend told you they were giving up bananas for January. Would you think, "There's someone who's in control of their bananas?" Or would you think, "Golly! I didn't know he had a banana problem."

And what kind of reason is "It's not doing me any harm" for

doing anything? A lot of people enjoy yoga. Have you ever heard a friend explain why she goes to yoga by saying, "It doesn't do me any harm?" The same applies to all genuine pleasures. It would be a silly thing to say. When it comes to drinking, though, it's even more silly to say it doesn't do you any harm, because everybody knows it does!

A PROBLEM WAITING TO HAPPEN

Here's a question for you: If you believe there is such a thing as a happy "normal" drinker, why are you not one already? All you have to do is drink less.

If it could be fixed so that you could drink just once a week for the rest of your life, would you accept it? Better still, if it was made possible for you to control your drinking so that you did it only when you really wanted to, that would be pretty exciting, wouldn't it?

But that's what you already do!

Every time you've had a drink you've done so because you wanted to, even though part of your brain wished you didn't. So you think you'd be happier if you only drank once a week? Well, do it then! What's stopping you? You've had every opportunity to be a once-a-week drinker, but you haven't taken it. Why?

Could it be that you wouldn't have been happy drinking just once a week?

Of course you wouldn't. Neither is any other drinker. Sure, there are drinkers who can discipline themselves to just one a week, but can you really believe that any of them are happy restricting themselves every day for the whole of their lives? Remember,

THE TENDENCY IS TO DRINK MORE, NOT LESS

"Normal" drinkers are constantly repressing the urge to drink more. They are still laboring under the illusion that drinking is an escape and a relief. All it takes is a trauma of some kind for them to increase their drinking in the belief that it will provide some comfort.

We meet plenty of people who have developed alcohol problems in their 30s or 40s, or even later. They have all spent their lives believing that drinking could give them some pleasure or crutch, but their desire to drink was never enough to outweigh their knowledge of the dangers or the discipline they used to restrict their intake. One trauma was all it took to tip the balance.

ANYONE WHO BELIEVES ALCOHOL PROVIDES SOME SORT OF PLEASURE OR CRUTCH, WHETHER THEY DRINK OR NOT, IS IN DANGER OF HAVING A DRINK PROBLEM

We've established that the problem of addiction is not with the drinker but with the drink. How can the same drug be beneficial for one group of people and devastating for another? That's like saying the rain that comes in through one missing roof tile is better than the rain that comes in through two.

Alcohol doesn't benefit anybody except the industry that

peddles it. There is no demarcation line between "normal" drinking and problem drinking; it is all part of the same disease. The problem drinker is just at a more advanced stage.

When you began this book you may have been hoping it would put you in a position where you could drink casually like all the "normal" drinkers you know. You should now understand that there is no place for half measures: Cutting down is not an option. Every "normal" drinker is a problem drinker waiting to happen.

Just as the only way to stop the rain coming in is to repair the hole in the roof, the only way to get free from the alcohol trap is to stop drinking. The choice is yours: Quit completely or stay forever in the trap.

SUMMARY

- Alcohol is useful as an antiseptic, a detergent, and a fuel. It has no other benefits whatsoever
- "Normal" drinkers only appear to be in control because they are oblivious to the trap they're in
- Cutting down always results in drinking more
- "Normal" drinkers can't describe the pleasure they get from drinking. That's because there is no pleasure
- "Normal" drinking and problem drinking are just different stages of the same disease

CHAPTER 13

CLOSING QUESTIONS

You are entering the final stages before releasing yourself from the alcohol trap. It's time to remove any lingering doubts that you might have.

Very soon you are going to experience an exhilarating sense of freedom. Your mindset now should be like that of someone about to make a parachute jump. You've been through a proper and proven course of instruction; you've prepared yourself mentally; you're confident that everything you've been taught is correct; and you've boarded the plane expecting a wonderfully liberating experience, but it's completely understandable that, as you stand by the door of the plane getting ready to jump, you feel the butterflies in your stomach.

If we were purely logical beings, we would have no fear of parachute jumps because all the data would tell us it's safe. Yet we still get the butterflies—that's completely natural. Any lingering concerns you might have about quitting drinking for good are also completely natural. By now you should be absolutely clear that drinking does nothing for you whatsoever, that you only think it gives you pleasure or a crutch because you've been caught in the cycle of addiction and that's how addictive drugs work. If you are not clear about this, please go back and reread the relevant chapters. If you are, it is still likely that you will be experiencing feelings of apprehension. That's only natural. Call it the fear of the unknown. Keep in mind that this is where the comparison to a parachute jump ends. In reality, rather than jumping from an aircraft thousands of feet above the ground, you're simply stepping through an open door on to solid ground, into a world of light, sunshine, blue sky, and fresh air.

WHEN WILL I KNOW I'VE KICKED IT?

With any nerve-wracking experience, the first thing we want to know is when it will end. Because of the brainwashing, problem drinkers are afraid that they will have to go through some terrible ordeal in order to quit, or that life will never be enjoyable again after they have. They expect to suffer and so they want to know when the suffering will end.

• When you can go a whole day without drinking?

• When you can go a week?

• When you can enjoy social events without alcohol?

All these suggestions assume that you will start off with a feeling of sacrifice or deprivation. If you do, there's no telling how long that feeling will last.

For you, it's different this time. You don't need to worry. With Easyway,

YOU BECOME A NONDRINKER AS SOON AS YOU FINISH YOUR FINAL DRINK

You may have already decided that you've had your final drink. Even though we ask you not to make any change to your drinking while you read the book, some people vow never to drink again before they start reading this book. Others stop drinking along the way because they just have no desire to do it any more. It doesn't matter when you do it: What is crucial is that you are left in no doubt that it is, or was, your final drink.

It's not the one you *think* will be your last, or the one you *hope* will be your last; when you quit with Easyway, there is no doubt. Get it clearly into your mind: You won't miss drinking; in fact you will enjoy life infinitely more and be far better equipped to cope with stress when you're free.

THE ENDLESS TORTURE OF THE WILLPOWER METHOD

People who quit with the willpower method are always waiting for some sign of confirmation that they're free.

They also spend their time suspecting that there could be bad news lurking just around the corner. It's like a dark shadow stalking their every move.

A woman suspects she might have a terminal disease, so she goes for tests and is told that she will have to wait months or years for the result. Imagine the torture—hoping for good news, fearing bad news, and spending every day worrying because she simply doesn't know for certain which it will be. Now put yourself in her position and imagine you had to wait the rest of your life for those results. That's what it's like for people who are not certain they've kicked drinking completely. They spend the rest of their lives waiting for something that they hope will never happen.

CAN I REALLY BE CURED COMPLETELY?

There is nothing stupid or unusual in believing that stopping drinking will be incredibly hard. You've been subjected to this belief all your life and it has been reinforced by any attempt you made, and many others you may have observed being made, to quit using the willpower method. That desperate craving you got when you tried not to drink may have gone against everything you told yourself about the evils of alcohol, but the craving was very real and so is the irritability and misery you felt when you tried to use willpower to stop. Don't expect to feel the same way again.

When we're forced to consider drinking logically, we can

easily accept that it is harmful to us, yet we still feel a desire to do it. This is utterly confusing and we assume that we must get some tremendous boost from it that outweighs the harmful effects. The fact that we can't put our finger on what this boost is and don't understand the desire doesn't mean it's difficult to understand. The only reason we don't understand it is because we've been brainwashed with false information about it. Just as you would struggle to understand arithmetic if you'd been taught incorrectly, you can see that the information you've been fed doesn't add up, but you have no idea how to make sense of the problem. The great news is that this is not a challenging arithmetic problem to solve. It's as simple as 1+1+1+1=4.

The truth is very simple to understand:

- the desire to drink comes from the Big Monster—the brainwashing since birth that drinking gives us some kind of pleasure or crutch

- the Little Monster is physical withdrawal from alcohol; it was created when we started drinking. It's actually incredibly mild, almost imperceptible

- the slight anxiety we feel when we're without a drink is merely the Little Monster wanting its fix, but it triggers the Big Monster which creates a feeling of deprivation. It's a thought process that creates unpleasant feelings, not the physical withdrawal

• the Little Monster was created by drinking in the first place. Therefore, drinking does not relieve the anxiety, panic, and feeling of deprivation; it causes it

Get this straight in your mind and it's easy to see that if you remove the cause of the anxiety, you will start to enjoy life immediately, free from drinking.

The willpower method requires you to fight through the anxiety, rather than removing it. Quitting becomes a battle and in the first few days, when your willpower is at its strongest, you will have the upper hand. Over time, though, your willpower will weaken and the Little Monster's cries to be fed will get louder and louder. At this point you start to feel victory slipping from your grasp.

Now the battle creeps in: One half of your mind is determined to be a nondrinker, the other keeps urging you to drink. Is it surprising that we get so confused, irritable, and miserable on the willpower method? It would be a miracle if we didn't!

Even if you can muster enough willpower to kill the Little Monster, without destroying the Big Monster you will always remain vulnerable to the temptation to drink.

With Easyway you kill the Big Monster first. In other words, you unravel the brainwashing and see alcohol for what it really is: a poison that controls and debilitates everybody who takes it. You understand how you were fooled into believing that it was a pleasure or a crutch, and so you remove all desire for it. When you come to kill the Little Monster, you find it is no ordeal at all. In fact, you can enjoy the process, knowing that you are destroying a mortal enemy.

UNDERSTAND THAT THE BIG MONSTER TRIGGERS A THOUGHT PROCESS AND THAT YOU CAN NOW CORRECT THAT THOUGHT PROCESS

JUST THE ONE

A question we are often asked at our centers is, "Once I'm cured, will I be able to have the odd glass?" The answer is simple: "Why would you want to?" If you approach your final drink still thinking that you'd like to have the odd drink now and again, you haven't followed all the instructions and the Big Monster still lurks in your mind.

There will be times when you are tested. Other drinkers who don't understand the alcohol trap will see how confident and in control you are as a nondrinker and will assume the odd one won't set you back. What these drinkers don't understand is that you have absolutely no desire to have just the one. But you understand it.

With AA or the willpower method, you are told that one drink is all it will take to trap you again so you have to spend the rest of your life fighting it. With Easyway, you have no more desire to have one drink than you do to take arsenic.

CAN LIFE REALLY BE FUN WITHOUT ALCOHOL?

Drinkers are all afraid that if they take drinking out of their lives, they will take out the enjoyment too. It's easy to see why that would stop you from trying to quit. Nobody wants to lead a joyless life, devoid of laughter and excitement. But why should you think life without alcohol is devoid of laughter and excitement? Was life like that before you started drinking?

Drinking actually reduces your ability to find the pleasure and excitement in life. It deadens your senses, messes up your judgment, warps your self-awareness so you think you're being interesting when you're not, makes you vulnerable and insecure, and often makes you sick. If you really want to suck all the juice out of life, surely it's better to remain lucid and alert and keep your body functioning perfectly.

We're brainwashed into a romanticized view of drinking. Often the things we think we'll miss are things we haven't even experienced for real. Where we do remember fun occasions involving alcohol, there will be other aspects that actually made it enjoyable, such as the company, the food, the setting, the entertainment, or something worth celebrating.

Now, replace any thoughts that such occasions won't be enjoyable again without alcohol with the realization that you'll now be able to enjoy them more because you won't be rendered physically and mentally incapable by alcohol, you won't be suffering the restlessness of always craving a drink, and you won't have the misery of knowing you're an addict. On the contrary, you'll have the added joy of knowing you're not!

In most situations we're not even aware of how we feel while we're drinking. The only time we're really aware of how alcohol makes us feel is when we want to drink but can't, or we're drinking but wish we didn't have to. In both cases it makes us miserable.

TAKE AWAY THE DRINKING AND YOU REMOVE THE MISERY

HOW WILL I COPE IN A CRISIS?

We've said a lot about the myth that alcohol gives you pleasure, but what about the belief that it provides a crutch to help you through difficult times? The brainwashing on this subject is so strong, even lifelong nondrinkers have been conditioned to turn to drink in times of stress.

Say you do try to escape a stressful situation by gazing into the bottom of a glass for a while. It doesn't matter what's causing your stress—a family row, pressure at work, financial difficulties—the problem is that eventually you have to return to the real world. The drink hasn't made the problem go away; in fact, it's gotten worse because it's been left to fester.

Have you ever found yourself in the middle of a domestic row and thought, "It doesn't matter that we're shouting horrible things at one another and that it's really painful because I can just go and drink and it will be all right?" Or did the fact that you drink make the row worse? Perhaps it even caused the row in the first place.

ALCOHOL REDUCES YOUR ABILITY TO COPE WITH STRESSFUL SITUATIONS AND ADDS TO THE STRESS

There will be stressful situations in life. We all have to go through them whether we drink or not, and the stronger we are, mentally and physically, the better equipped we'll be to deal with them. If you believe that alcohol provides a crutch in these situations, then the next time a stressful situation arises after you've quit your first thought will be, "At times like this I would have had a drink to calm down," and you will feel deprived that you can no longer do so.

Accept that there will be ups and downs in life after you've quit and prepare yourself mentally, so that you don't fall into the trap. Be ready to remind yourself that any stress you feel is not because you can't drink and that the stress will pass more easily because you don't drink.

You're stronger now. You don't have the added stress of being a slave to alcohol and you're better equipped to tackle the inevitable stresses of life rather than burying your head in the sand. It's a win–win situation.

BEING FREE FROM ALCOHOL ENHANCES ALL SITUATIONS IN LIFE—GOOD TIMES BECOME EVEN BETTER AND BAD TIMES ARE HANDLED MORE EASILY

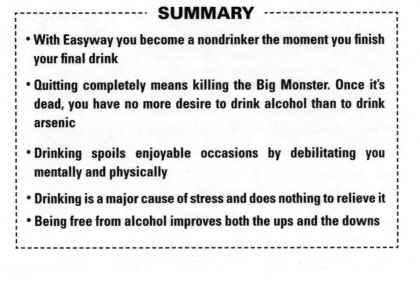

SUMMARY

- With Easyway you become a nondrinker the moment you finish your final drink

- Quitting completely means killing the Big Monster. Once it's dead, you have no more desire to drink alcohol than to drink arsenic

- Drinking spoils enjoyable occasions by debilitating you mentally and physically

- Drinking is a major cause of stress and does nothing to relieve it

- Being free from alcohol improves both the ups and the downs

Chapter 14

REPLACE FEAR WITH EXCITEMENT

Once you have removed the brainwashing, the next step is to replace all the negatives with the wonderful positives of being free.

When was the last time you woke up in the morning full of excitement and eager to get up and get on with the day? People in the alcohol trap tend to wake up with a sense of foreboding, a fear that something bad is going to happen, or is already happening, and they can't do anything about it. That fear is caused by alcohol. One of the great benefits of getting free is throwing off this constant dread and rediscovering the genuine joy of life.

We explained in Chapter Eight that the fear is like the anxiety that long-term convicts feel when they finally get released. It's a lack of confidence in their ability to cope with the world around them and an inability to see the genuine pleasures that are there for them. A famous example is the character Brooks in *The Shawshank Redemption*, played wonderfully by James Whitmore. Brooks has been in prison for 50 years. You would think that finally getting out after all that time would be the most ecstatic feeling in the world. But Brooks finds it a miserable experience and ends up hanging himself.

It's a tragedy, and one of the most upsetting scenes of a brilliant movie. You want to put your arm around Brooks and show him all the terrific things that life has to offer when you're free. Meet friends, go for a walk, have a nice meal, go to the movies… Brooks' mind has been altered by prison. When you're denied all the usual pleasures in life, your idea of pleasure changes. On the outside, he needs help in recognizing genuine pleasures and being made to believe they are for him. Tragically, Brooks never gets that help. But you can.

Alcohol addiction is like a prison. You lose the ability to enjoy the things you enjoyed before you started drinking. The alcohol-induced illusion of pleasure takes the place of genuine pleasures and becomes all you care about. You end up living for an illusion. The genuine pleasures still exist and they are still enjoyable, but as a drinker you always credited booze. Remember those fantastic nights out, with the people that you love, the amazing shows, parties, and laughs that you've had. At the time you gave all the credit for those good times to alcohol. You just need to have your eyes opened and see things as they really are.

The beauty of Easyway is that it not only helps you escape the prison, but it also changes your mindset in the process, so you are able to enjoy genuine pleasures from the minute you first get free. In fact, many people find they get that feeling of excitement back before they have their final drink because they know for certain that they are about to get free and they can't wait to start enjoying life without alcohol. You won't be missing out on anything.

A WONDERFUL ACHIEVEMENT

When you started reading Chapter One and we told you that you had to read the whole book in order and not skip ahead, you probably felt a twinge of frustration. You were eager to get to the bit you'd been dreaming of—the cure! In spite of your skepticism you still had a sense of excitement at the prospect of getting free. Now you understand that the whole book is the cure. You've followed the instructions and now stand on the brink of achieving something amazing: You are about to become a happy nondrinker.

Congratulate yourself on this achievement and let the excitement build inside you. You used to have doubts about ever getting free—now you know that escape is in the palm of your hand. Remind yourself that there is no reason to feel miserable; on the contrary, you have every reason to feel elated. But you may be still feeling the effects of your drinking and struggling to convince yourself that this is going to be as easy as I say. Let's just take a deep breath and look at the whole picture rationally.

FINISH UNRAVELING THE ILLUSIONS

The fear of life without drinking is caused by myths, illusions, and brainwashing. Addiction traps you by turning logic on its head.

We've looked at these illusions closely and shown that they have no bearing on reality. In fact, they tend to be the opposite of reality. Until we realize that they are illusions, we go through life without trying to unravel them and assume that they are real, but as soon as it's pointed out to us that they are illusions, it's easy to see through them to the truth. Easyway exposes the myths and illusions, reverses the brainwashing, and helps you to see through it all.

Any lingering fears you have that stopping will not be easy are merely the result of brainwashing.

You've been brainwashed into believing that drinking gives you some sort of pleasure or support and that stopping is hard. You have come a long way in unraveling that brainwashing; now you need to finish the job.

THE FEAR OF STOPPING DRINKING IS CREATED BY DRINKING

TAKE AWAY THE DRINK AND THE FEAR GOES TOO

ACHIEVING CERTAINTY

As soon as you get free from the alcohol trap, you'll look back with wonder at how easy it was to escape. You'll be amazed at how good you feel and your only regret will be not having made your escape sooner.

At the moment you may still feel like someone struggling to get out of a deep pit, but once you get out you'll realize there was no pit. All you had to do was take a step forward instead of a step back. Clear doubt from your mind—you are on the verge of something AMAZING!

We are sometimes asked, "How can you know for certain that something will *not* happen?" In other words, even if you do manage to quit, how can you be sure you won't fall into the trap again? After all, the chances of being struck by a meteorite are infinitesimally small, yet nobody can say with absolute certainty that it will never happen to them.

That's very true, but let's take a different example. What are the odds of you getting eaten by a shark? Well, that depends on several things, not least of which is whether you ever go in the sea. If you never go in the sea, it's safe to say you will never get eaten by a shark.

The same degree of certainty applies when you escape the alcohol trap.

If you never drink again, it's guaranteed that you won't fall back into the alcohol trap. When you escape with Easyway and have no desire to drink, you know with absolute certainty that you will never drink again.

Let go of your preconceptions and allow the true picture to take shape in your mind. The key to seeing through any illusion is not through willpower; it is through understanding and correcting your beliefs and seeing it as it really is. So relax, open your mind, and enjoy getting free.

NO GOING BACK

Once you get it into your head that it's just fear that prevents drinkers from stopping, you may be tempted to try and allay that fear by telling yourself you can always start drinking again if it gets too hard—that quitting doesn't have to be final.

If you start off with that attitude, you're very likely to fail, because you have allowed doubts to remain in your mind. Instead, start off with the certainty that you're going to be free forever. To achieve that certainty, you have to allow your mind to free itself of all doubt and let go of the desire to drink.

STEP FORWARD

It's time to start taking the practical forward steps that will see you become a happy nondrinker for life. When you first picked up this book, you had a choice: You could have continued to bury your head in the sand and stumble further and further into the miserable slavery of drinking, but you chose to take positive action to resolve your problem. All you need to do is keep making positive choices.

There are three very important facts to keep in mind:

1. Alcohol does absolutely nothing for you at all.
It is crucial that you understand why this is so and accept it, so that you never feel you're being deprived.

2. There is no need for a transitional period.

Often referred to as the "withdrawal period," it is widely assumed that this is an essential part of any addiction cure, but with Easyway you have no need to wait for anything. The moment you stop drinking is the moment you become free.

3. There is no such thing as "just the one."

One drink is enough to make you a drinker and must be seen for what it is: part of a lifelong chain of self-destruction. People who see that there is no benefit in drinking have no desire to do so, not even "just the once," and therefore run no risk of falling back into the trap.

YOUR MORTAL ENEMY

Why would anyone regard something that's destroying them as a friend? That's what a nondrinker would think. Yet when drinkers, gamblers, smokers, heroin users, and other addicts try to quit by willpower, they feel they're losing a friend. They grieve for their "loss," becoming even more miserable than when they were drinking.

Imagine living under an evil tyrant, who brutalizes your people and keeps you living in fear. How would you feel if one day you were suddenly rid of this tyrant? Would you grieve? Would you mope?

Of course you wouldn't; you would rejoice. Alcohol is not your friend; it's your mortal enemy, so rejoice and get ready to celebrate for the rest of your life. From the moment you quit, every time you think about alcohol you will rejoice that it no longer has you enslaved.

That's the beauty about quitting with Easyway: You don't have to put drinking out of your mind. Remember, Easyway doesn't help you to resist the temptation to drink; it removes the temptation altogether. So you can think about drinking all you like because every time you do you will be able to rejoice in that wonderful feeling of being free.

People who try to resist the temptation to drink by not thinking about it put themselves through mental torture because whenever you try not to think about something, you can be sure that it's the one thing that you can't get out of your mind. Try it for yourself —don't think about elephants. Now, what's the first thing that comes into your head?

THINK READY

During the first few days after your final drink, the Little Monster will still be alive and it will be grumbling away, sending increasingly desperate messages to your brain that it wants you to interpret as "I need a drink." That thought might even pop into your mind, but don't panic. Thoughts don't count; it's what we do with those thoughts that counts. If you think, "I can't have one" or "I mustn't have one," then you'll be miserable. You'll be moping after an illusion, something that doesn't even exist. But if you think, "YIPPEE I'M FREE!" you'll feel wonderful. And the more you think about it, the more wonderful you'll feel.

So relax, accept any slight discomfort for what it really is— the death throes of the Little Monster—and remind yourself, "Non-drinkers don't have this problem. This is a feeling that drinkers suffer all their lives. It's caused by alcohol. Isn't it great? It will soon be gone forever."

THE WITHDRAWAL PANGS WILL BECOME MOMENTS OF PLEASURE

There may well be times during the first few days in particular when you forget you've quit. You think, "I'll have a drink," and then you remember with joy that you're now a nondrinker. But you wonder why the thought entered your head. You were convinced you'd reversed the brainwashing. If you're not prepared for this, doubts can creep in and you may start to question your decision to quit.

Prepare yourself for such moments now, so that when they occur you remain calm and use them as a reminder of the wonderful freedom you've gained. The associations that you've always made with drinking, such as seeing friends, eating out, going to parties, etc., can linger on after the Little Monster has died and catch you unawares, but occasionally forgetting that you no longer drink isn't a bad sign; it's a very good one. It's proof that your life is returning to the happy state you were in before you got hooked on alcohol, when your whole existence wasn't dominated by the drug.

When you're prepared for these moments, they will actually come as a pleasant reminder, rather than a nasty surprise. Instead of instilling doubt and making you think, "I can't do this," you will respond by thinking, "Isn't it great! I'm free!"

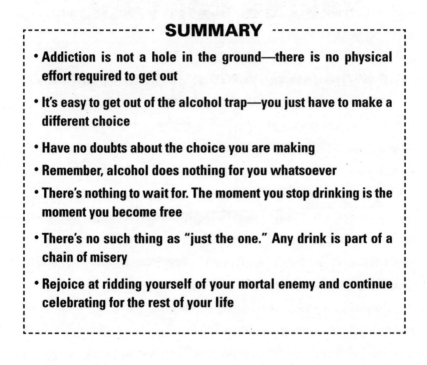

SUMMARY

- Addiction is not a hole in the ground—there is no physical effort required to get out

- It's easy to get out of the alcohol trap—you just have to make a different choice

- Have no doubts about the choice you are making

- Remember, alcohol does nothing for you whatsoever

- There's nothing to wait for. The moment you stop drinking is the moment you become free

- There's no such thing as "just the one." Any drink is part of a chain of misery

- Rejoice at ridding yourself of your mortal enemy and continue celebrating for the rest of your life

TAKING CONTROL

When you can recognize the trap you're in, it's easy to see what you need to do to take control of your drinking.

Everyone has their own reasons for wanting to stop drinking. Health is the most common one. Perhaps you've started to feel an aching around the kidneys, or you can't sleep, or you keep getting headaches, or you're fed up with feeling constantly tired and hungover, or old before your time. The alarm bells have started ringing, and so you've decided it's time for action.

Money is another common reason given for quitting. When you add up what you spend on booze—it's not unusual for a problem drinker to squander $150,000 on alcohol in a lifetime—it only adds to your sense of stupidity. The way alcoholism makes you feel about yourself is a major cause of misery and this is exacerbated by another common reason for quitting, the social effects of drinking. The way alcohol affects your moods and behavior, and how that affects family and friends, can be devastating. If you're fortunate enough to recognize it before it's too late, then ending the damage you're doing to your relationships and the pain you're causing people you care about can provide a wonderful bonus. If you feel the damage to those areas of your life is already done, then don't despair: Whatever the future holds for you, you're infinitely better equipped to handle it as a nondrinker.

Drinkers are well aware of the many good reasons not to drink, but it's only when you succeed in stopping that you realize the greatest gain to be had from quitting: to escape from slavery.

The feeling of being controlled by an addiction is the main source of misery for drinkers. You wish you could stop, but you can't. You keep getting drawn back in by a feeble craving that you just can't seem to resist. You react as you react to other obstacles in life: by applying all your willpower. And when that doesn't work, you can only conclude that you're too weak and incapable to conquer this one problem. It's scary. With all hope of escape dashed, you close your mind to the terrible effects of being a drinker and surrender yourself to a life of miserable slavery.

That's why addicts often seem to be in wilful self-destruct mode; they've given up all hope of escape and their only option is denial. The tragedy is that they don't understand the trap they're in. If they did:

THEY WOULD FIND IT EASY TO BE FREE

Thinking about the downsides of drinking doesn't help set you free; if that was the case, you would have escaped long ago.

WE DON'T DRINK TO EXERCISE POWER OVER REASON; WE DRINK BECAUSE WE'RE POWERLESS

Those reasons are phoney, a trick played by the Big Monster, and until you remove them, focusing on all the reasons not to drink is only going to add to your misery.

When you understand the trap you're in, you can see why the willpower method doesn't work and what you need to do to take control. When you succeed in stopping, you will look back on your days as a drinker and rejoice in your newfound freedom— the freedom to look at other drinkers, not with envy or a feeling of deprivation but with pity and compassion. You won't envy them; they will envy you!

The greatest gain to be made from becoming a nondrinker is not the good health, the money, or the social stability—although they are fantastic bonuses—but to no longer feel like a pathetic, doomed slave. That's the freedom that all drinkers wish they could attain.

YOUR FAVORITE TIPPLE?

What's your poison? This old-fashioned phrase touches on one of the ingenious illusions of the alcohol trap, and one that is relentlessly pushed by the alcohol peddlers: that drinkers are discerning in their choice of drink. The snobbery and pretentiousness surrounding wine and whiskey would be hilarious if it wasn't so deadly. Wine buffs will gather and talk nonsense for hours on end about grape varieties and soil structures and climate etc., anything to distract them from the fact that they're pouring large quantities of poison down their throats.

Whiskey connoisseurs talk about the characteristic flavors of peat and brine. Can you think of anything more disgusting than swallowing earth or sea water! And these days we're even expected to look for the subtle nuances in lager!

It's a clever trick being played by the drinks industry. The image of "the discerning connoisseur" is designed to keep you in the trap by deluding you into thinking you are in control. You're not just throwing any old poison down your throat; you're making an educated choice.

WISE UP!

Whatever pretentious nonsense it says on the label, it's still poison. The only discerning choice to make is the choice not to drink it. Only when it comes to this decision do drinkers become aware that they are not, in fact, in control. They are very familiar with all the powerful reasons not to drink, yet they feel powerless to resist the urge.

When you're in the alcohol trap, you're pulled in opposite directions. Part of your brain is telling you not to drink, but another part is compelling you to keep drinking. It leaves you in a constant state of confusion: If you want to stop, why can't you just stop? With anything else in life, you know that if you wanted to stop and had very good reasons to do so, you would stop, easily and immediately, so why can't you apply the same control to drinking?

The answer is simple:

YOU DON'T CONTROL ALCOHOL; ALCOHOL CONTROLS YOU

WHO'S PULLING THE STRINGS?

Perhaps you find this confusing. After all, didn't I say earlier in the book that nobody has ever forced you to drink; it has always been you making that choice? And yet now we're saying you're not in control as long as you drink. How can someone who is not in control exercise a choice?

Have you ever been to a hypnotist's show? People are called up on stage and made to do ridiculous things for the audience's amusement. Those poor, humiliated guinea pigs are not forced to perform ridiculous acts; they choose to do them. But their choice is manipulated by the hypnotist.

Addiction controls you in the same way. It makes you think you're making choices of your own free will but, in fact, you're being controlled. Your choices are not based on reality; they're based on illusions. And the control begins from the moment you have your first drink.

This constant wrestling match between logic and illusion is

what goes on in every addict's mind. It's confusing and makes us feel foolish and weak. Your understanding of the alcohol trap means you can now see that the only way to make controlled choices is to stop drinking, but the addict who is controlled by alcohol doesn't see stopping as an option.

As long as anyone goes on believing that they're in control of their drinking, they will fail to do the one thing that will cure their problem: stop drinking. Only when you understand and accept that alcohol controls you, not the other way round, can you see that the only way to change this situation is not to drink.

It isn't just the only way; it's the easy way. Go on insisting that you are in control and you will continue to make life hard for yourself. You will be pushing against the wrong side of the door. This is how willpower keeps you in the trap. With the willpower method you preserve the belief that you can control alcohol, and by doing so you sentence yourself to a lifetime of hardship. Let go of that illusion, accept that alcohol has made you a slave, and escape will be easy.

USING THE KEY

Cunning and ingenious though it is, the alcohol trap has one fatal flaw: As the prisoner, you hold the key to your own release. In order to escape, you just need three things to happen:

1. You must recognize that you're in a trap.

2. You must recognize that you hold the key.

3. You must be shown how to use the key.

Only Easyway does this for you. Everything you've read so far has been designed to help you see the trap you're in and recognize that you hold the key.

1. The trap is the addiction.

2. The key is unraveling the brainwashing that keeps you addicted—killing the Big Monster.

3. The final step is to turn the key—to kill the Little Monster —and walk free.

These are the three steps to taking control of your drink problem. So let's make sure that steps 1 and 2 have been fully accomplished.

We've explained about the alcohol trap and how it keeps you hooked by creating the illusion of pleasure. You should be completely clear that any pleasure or crutch you thought you got from alcohol was merely an illusion created by brainwashing. You should be in no doubt that alcohol does nothing for you whatsoever: It doesn't give you courage, nor does it take away fear. It doesn't make you more interesting or entertaining, nor does it help you to be calm. It's not a reward; it's pure punishment. If you have any lingering doubts about any of these points, go back to Chapter 7 and read on from there.

If you are completely clear on all these points, then the Big

Monster should be gone from your mind. You should also be clear that the only way to control alcohol is not to drink. Cutting down or just having "the odd one" is not the best of both worlds; it's the worst of both worlds. As long as you put alcohol in your system, alcohol will control you.

THE ONLY PEOPLE WHO ARE NOT CONTROLLED BY ALCOHOL ARE NONDRINKERS

You become a nondrinker the moment you stop drinking without any desire ever to drink again.

From that moment the Little Monster will begin to die. This is the final step. Congratulations on reaching this point. Everything you do from now should be a celebration of your freedom from slavery to alcohol.

SHARING YOUR SECRET

Keeping a drink problem to yourself is not easy but neither is sharing it with others. Drinking traps you in a very stressful limbo as you go to great lengths to cover up your secret. When you're ready to take control of your problem, you will feel more confident about telling other people what you've been through, but there are always concerns. You might be afraid that people will be angry and will lose respect for you. People who love and trust you will almost certainly be hurt, but they will also respect you for tackling your problem and will want to help.

It's also very likely that the people you think you've been deceiving haven't been deceived at all. They'll have noticed the change in your behavior and may already have been affected by it. The longer you go on trying to deceive them, the more these feelings will grow into distrust and dislike. Own up and you give them the opportunity to understand why your behavior has changed and to help you sort it out. Don't be surprised to find that they are relieved by your admission.

You're the best person to judge when the time is right to share the truth. You may feel right now that your loved ones are not ready for the full story of your alcohol addiction and that "dumping it on them" would be unfair. That's fine. Once you're free and enjoying the confidence and self-respect that come with it, you'll be better equipped to work out the best way to come clean.

Don't panic: If you want to quietly and discreetly become a happy nondrinker without making some kind of announcement, then that is perfectly fine. The most important person on this planet is you! Do what you feel is right for you.

ENJOY BREAKING FREE

You're ready to kill the Little Monster and make your escape from the alcohol trap. Remember, you have nothing to fear from stopping, only terrific gains to make. Any fear you might feel is just the last-minute nerves of the parachutist. Remember, there is no huge leap; you are walking to freedom. Fear is not relieved by drinking; it's caused by it. You are the lucky fly on the wall of the pitcher plant that is being given the power to fly free. Take it!

See yourself as a nondrinker would see you. You know that alcohol does absolutely nothing for you whatsoever. You also know that it is a poison that causes untold harm. You can stop the damage immediately by never drinking again. You have nothing to lose and everything to gain. Think about Brooks in *The Shawshank Redemption*. Imagine that's you, struggling to see the genuine pleasures in life and fearful that they're not for you. Put your arm around your shoulder and remind yourself of all the fantastic advantages there are to being free:

• Good health

• More balanced moods

• Better relationships

• Higher self-esteem

• Less stress

- Better sleep

- Better concentration

- Clearer thinking

- More choice over how you spend your time

- More money

- More fun

- More stamina

- Less worry

And most important of all

CONTROL OVER YOUR LIFE

Very soon you will make a solemn vow that you will never drink alcohol again. Before you get to that wonderful moment, there is one final stage that you need to prepare for. We've told you that with Easyway there is no need for a painful withdrawal period, but we've also said that the Little Monster doesn't die as soon as you stop drinking. So what happens during those first few days after your final drink, when all traces of alcohol are disappearing from your body? The next chapter explains the truth about withdrawal.

SUMMARY

- The biggest benefit of stopping drinking is ending the slavery
- See through the illusion of "discerning drinking." You don't control alcohol; alcohol controls you
- Addiction deludes you into making harmful choices
- The only way to regain control over alcohol is to stop drinking
- You're ready to kill the Little Monster. Rejoice!

Chapter 16

THE TRUTH ABOUT WITHDRAWAL

IN THIS CHAPTER

•*A COMMON MISCONCEPTION* •*THE PANIC FEELING*
•*THE SYMPTOMS OF WITHDRAWAL*
•*WITHDRAWAL THROUGH WILLPOWER* •*ENJOYING THE FEELING*
•*NOTHING TO WAIT FOR* •*READY TO JUMP*

The time it takes for the Little Monster to die is a daunting period for drinkers who quit with the willpower method. With Easyway, it is a pleasure.

There is a common misconception among drinkers and non-drinkers that coming off the booze means going through a painful withdrawal period. As all the toxins leave your body, so the theory goes, you suffer a severe physical reaction. You will have heard of delirium tremens—the DTs—and other feverish symptoms that afflict withdrawing alcoholics. This belief is enough to prevent a lot of drinkers from even trying to quit. As with all the other reasons drinkers give for not stopping, it is a myth.

We've talked a lot about the restless feeling drinkers get when the alcohol is leaving their body and the Little Monster cries out for more, a feeling that is so slight as to be almost imperceptible.

Perhaps you've assumed that there's something different about the withdrawal you go through when you quit for good.

There isn't.

For most drinkers who quit there are no abnormal physical symptoms during withdrawal: no sweats or shakes, no headaches or palpitations. We only think we have to go through some terrible trauma because stopping on the willpower method can be psychological torture and that can itself create physical symptoms. We've explained that addiction is 1 percent physical and 99 percent mental. Every night, millions of drinkers manage to sleep soundly for eight hours and when they wake up they feel no pain after having to go so long without their drug. If the physical effects of withdrawal were so bad, it would wake them up in the night, desperate for a drink. In truth, most drinkers manage to last well into the day before they have their first drink. Until that point they've not only got by quite happily without any physical pain, they've not even been aware of any discomfort.

Now, if you were to stand in the way of them having that first drink they might well react as if you'd stamped on their toe, but that's not a reaction to physical pain; it's panic at the prospect of being deprived. When they're confident again of having that next drink, this panic subsides. If it were a physical pain, like toothache, it would be there all the time.

AVOIDING PANIC

You've probably experienced the panic feeling yourself. Most problem drinkers have. It's the panic that sets in when you don't know where your next drink is coming from. Drinkers will go to great lengths to make sure they have a stock of booze so they know they're not going to be denied the opportunity to drink. Sneaking out of the house, lying about where you're going, borrowing money from strangers, even putting yourself in dangerous situations—it's all common behavior designed to avoid the panic feeling.

You do occasionally meet a heavy drinker who claims not to know the panic feeling. Hand on heart, they claim never to have experienced the panic of not knowing where their next drink is going to come from. A little further investigation explains why: They're so frightened of finding themselves in that position that they take every precaution to make sure it never happens!

Every drinker who is denied the opportunity to drink when they expect to experiences the panic feeling and this is the basis of any unpleasant withdrawal symptoms you might have heard about when people quit.

THOSE TERRIBLE SYMPTOMS

So just how serious can withdrawal get? The symptoms we keep hearing about are:

- **Anxiety**

- **Irritability**

- **Mood swings**

- **Nervousness**

- **Depression**

- **Confusion**

But wait a minute! These are not physical symptoms; they're psychological. What's more, they're symptoms that every drinker suffers to some degree WHILE THEY ARE DRINKING. These symptoms are brought on by alcohol, so the one way to ensure that you suffer them is to drink.

You may have read about the physical symptoms, such as:

- **Tiredness**

- **Headaches**

- **Stomach upsets**

- **Weak and aching muscles**

- **Heart palpitations**

- **The shakes**

- **The sweats**

• **The shivers**

• **Difficult breathing**

They look very much like the symptoms of flu, don't they? You may even have heard them described as such. Flu is not an uncommon ailment. You've probably had it several times in your life and no doubt expect to get it again. Does that thought make you panic? Flu is horrible; it can make you feel lousy, but it's not a pain you can't endure. If you could trade a week's flu for a lifetime of freedom from booze, wouldn't you take it?

Come to think of it, even if the withdrawal symptoms were painful, wouldn't you endure a little pain for a few days, in exchange for your freedom from slavery to alcohol? As a woman, you're very well equipped to endure pain. It's safe to say the pain of childbirth is many, many times worse than any natural discomfort a man has to endure in his life, but that doesn't put women off having babies. Pain is not the problem here; the problem is the fear and panic that pain induces if you don't understand why you're feeling it or what the consequences might be.

Take the mental reaction out of the picture and the symptoms of withdrawal from alcohol are nothing more than a slight restlessness, like an itch wanting to be scratched. Watch drinkers when they're denied the opportunity to drink. They'll be restless and fidgety. You'll notice little nervous tics and they'll be constantly doing things with their hands or grinding their teeth. This restlessness is triggered by an empty, insecure feeling, which can quickly turn into frustration AS A RESULT OF A THOUGHT PROCESS. "I want a drink," "I can't have one," "Arghhhhh!" That thought process creates a feeling of irritability, anxiety, anger, fear, and panic if they are not able to "satisfy" their alcohol craving.

You should be quite clear now that alcohol causes this feeling; it doesn't relieve it. As long as you understand that, you don't need to feel any sense of deprivation when you stop.

CONTINUE TO DRINK AND YOU'LL SUFFER THE RESTLESSNESS FOR THE REST OF YOUR LIFE

THE PAIN THRESHOLD

Pain only induces panic when you're not in control of it. Try pinching yourself and see how much you can endure before you have to stop. Now imagine that was someone else pinching you and think how you'd react. It's panic that makes us react long before we reach the limit of endurance.

If you go to the gym or an exercise class, you'll know that it can be painful when you really push yourself. Your muscles and lungs scream, but the feeling doesn't make you panic. You actually enjoy it because you know that you control it, plus it's an indication that you're doing yourself good.

WITHDRAWAL THROUGH WILLPOWER

It is the fear of being deprived that turns this slight restlessness into panic. You only feel deprived if you regard drinking as a pleasure or a crutch. When you have no desire to drink, the feeble cries of the Little Monster are barely perceptible and easily brushed off.

Imagine having a permanent itch that you're not allowed to scratch, added to which you believe the itch will last for the rest of your life unless you're allowed to scratch it. How long do you think you could last before your willpower gave in and you scratched the itch? If you did manage to hold out for a week or even more, imagine the relief you would feel when you finally gave in.

This is a description of the torture that drinkers go through when trying to quit with the willpower method. It's the Big Monster that gives you the urge to scratch the itch. Destroy the Big Monster and you can live with it quite happily until it disappears completely.

The problem for drinkers who quit with the willpower method is that for them the urge to scratch the itch does not die with the Little Monster. It is triggered by everything they ever associated with drinking, such as unwinding after a day's work, meeting friends, and going to parties. They think, "I used to drink on these occasions," and they still believe they're being deprived. The Big Monster is still alive, telling them that they need to scratch the itch.

The belief that drinking provides some sort of pleasure or crutch is a figment of the drinker's imagination, left over from the brainwashing. Drinking to satisfy this belief is like applying an ointment to a spot in the belief that it will clear it up, when all it does is to make the spot bigger and bigger. If you were in that situation and were told all you had to do was leave the spot for a few days and it would clear up on its own, you'd have no need or desire for the ointment.

It's easy to become a nondrinker when you realize that the empty, insecure feeling of wanting a drink is caused by the last drink you had, and that the one thing that will ensure you suffer that feeling for the rest of your life would be to drink another. You'll endure none of the suffering that you might have experienced in previous attempts because you will no longer believe you're being deprived. On the contrary, you'll experience a wonderful sense of freedom.

A POSITIVE SIGN

After your final drink you'll continue to experience the slight craving for a few days. This is not a physical pain; it's just the faint cries of the Little Monster wanting to be fed. Before you will have interpreted those cries as "I need a drink." Now you don't need to respond to them at all.

That doesn't mean you should ignore the feeling. Remember what we said at the end of Chapter 14 about trying *not* to think about something. It will dominate your thoughts. Use the faint cries of the Little Monster as a reminder of the wonderful change that is taking place. Keep in mind that the Little Monster was created when you first started drinking and it has continued to feed on every subsequent drink you've had. As soon as you stop drinking, you cut off the supply and that evil monster begins to die. In its death throes the Little Monster is trying to entice you to feed it. It may not be a pleasant feeling, but you can still take pleasure from it by using it to create a mental image of this parasite getting weaker and weaker and enjoy starving it to death.

Keep this mental image ready at all times and make sure you don't respond to its cries by thinking, "I need a drink." Drinking will only ensure that you continue to feel the empty, insecure feeling for the rest of your life.

Take a ruthless delight in feeling the Little Monster die. Even if you do get that feeling of "I need a drink" for a few days, don't worry about it. It's just the Little Monster doing everything it can to tempt you to feed it. As long as you're prepared for that, you will find it easy to keep starving it. You now have complete control over it. It's no longer destroying you; you are destroying it and soon you will be free forever.

NOTHING TO WAIT FOR?

The good news is that you can start enjoying the genuine pleasure of being a nondrinker from the moment you finish your final drink. There is nothing to wait for. Unlike drinkers who quit with the willpower method, you don't have to torture yourself waiting for something *not* to happen.

In most cases it takes just a few days for the Little Monster to die. During this period, people who use the willpower method tend to feel completely obsessed with being denied what they see as their pleasure or crutch, but then, after about three weeks, they suddenly realize that it's been a while since they thought about drinking. It's an exciting feeling… and a dangerous one.

One moment they believed that life would always be miserable without being able to drink; now they're convinced that time will solve their problem. They feel on top of the world. It's time to celebrate. What possible harm could it do to reward themselves with just one drink?

The fact that they even want that drink is proof that the Big Monster is still alive. They still believe that they've been depriving themselves. If they're foolish enough to go along with this belief and have a drink, they won't find it rewarding at all. There will be no illusion of pleasure because the illusion is caused by the partial relief of the symptoms of withdrawal. Now that they're no longer withdrawing, there is nothing to relieve.

Like a naughty child who has just opened a forbidden jar, they replace the lid and put the drink away, hoping that they've gotten away with it. They don't want their efforts to quit to be blown away so easily and for nothing. But that one drink is enough to revive the Little Monster and they have to draw on all their willpower to make sure they don't respond to the urge to drink again. But after a while the same thing happens. This time they can say to themselves, "I had a drink last time and didn't get hooked, so what harm can it do if I have another?" They're just wandering back into the trap.

Anyone who has tried to quit with the willpower method is likely to have experienced this scenario. With Easyway, when you realize you haven't thought about drinking for a while, your first thought is not to celebrate with a drink; it's

YIPPEE! I'M FREE! I DON'T HAVE TO DRINK ANY MORE!

With Easyway it doesn't matter how long it takes for the last symptoms of withdrawal to pass, you can relax and enjoy life from the moment you finish your final drink, confident that you don't ever have to go through the misery of alcohol addiction again.

Drinkers who quit with the willpower method never get to enjoy that certainty. The physical symptoms of withdrawal are easily confused with everyday pangs such as hunger and stress, so when they experience these everyday feelings they interpret them as "I need a drink." Drinking won't even partially relieve natural pangs like hunger, but their brainwashed mind is still convinced that it will help them relax. Their stress is increased because they believe that they're being deprived of a crutch that will ease the situation.

So what do they do: go through the rest of their life believing they're missing out, or find out for sure? There's only way to do that and that's to drink again. If they do, they find that their stress is not relieved by alcohol—in fact, it's increased by it, coupled with their sense of disappointment at having given in to temptation. Before you know it, they're drinking just as before.

READY TO JUMP?

Very soon you'll have your final drink and will make a solemn vow never to drink again. It's perfectly understandable if you're feeling the butterflies in your stomach. Just remind yourself of two simple facts:

- **The alcoholic drinks industry depends on fear to keep you hooked.**

- **Alcohol doesn't relieve the fear; it causes it.**

Unlike when you were in the trap, you now have control over your perception of drinking. Remind yourself that nothing bad is going to happen as a result of you stopping. On the contrary, you have many wonderful gains to make.

There is nothing unknown lying in wait for you.

What you are doing is something you've already done thousands of times before, every time you've drained your last glass at the end of the evening. This drink just happens to be a special one.

IT WILL BE YOUR VERY LAST!!

ALREADY STOPPED?

If you stopped drinking before you started reading this book and you're reluctant to drink again, that's fine, provided you are confident that you've killed the Big Monster and you have no doubts whatsoever that you are not making a sacrifice or depriving yourself in any way. Just confirm that you have had your last drink and make the vow.

Remember what you have to look forward to. In just a matter of days you'll feel stronger physically and mentally; you'll have more energy, more confidence, more self-respect, and more money. Don't put off this wonderful freedom, not for a week, a day, or even five seconds. There is nothing to wait for. You become a non-drinker the moment you finish your final drink.

Replace any last-minute nerves with a feeling of excitement as we go through the final checks before your jump.

REJOICE! YOU'RE ABOUT TO BE FREE!

SUMMARY

- You only feel unpleasant feelings with withdrawal if you think you're being deprived

- The discomfort is psychological, caused by panic. Without the desire to drink, there is no panic

- The physical symptoms are barely perceptible—recognize them as the death throes of the Little Monster and rejoice

- Be aware that everyday pangs such as hunger and stress feel the same as withdrawal, but drinking will not relieve them

- Drinkers suffer withdrawal pangs all the time. Nondrinkers don't suffer them at all

- Now that you're in control of your own mindset, feel the excitement of what you are about to achieve

YOUR CHECKLIST

Just a few checks as a failsafe before you step into your new life as a happy nondrinker.

What has been the greatest achievement of your life? Exam success? A career goal reached? When you quit drinking you will undoubtedly rank that achievement right up there with the best. Like all major achievements, it will have involved thorough preparation and dedication and you will not have gone into it without carrying out your final checks to make sure everything you've worked for is in place.

So, just to make sure you're properly prepared, let's run through a final check list.

1. FEEL EAGER AND EXCITED

You're now in control of your frame of mind. Make sure it's positive. Anticipate it as you would if you were about to escape from a miserable degrading prison. When that moment actually comes, it's more wonderful than you could ever have imagined. Put yourself in that frame of mind now. Anticipate a feeling more wonderful than you can imagine and tell yourself, "Great! I don't need to drink any more. I am about to free myself from misery and degradation. I can't wait!"

This is a time to rejoice. You're about to walk free from an evil trap that has kept you imprisoned and taken the joy out of life. It's time to reclaim the happiness you deserve and banish those feelings of misery, confusion, fear, and anger forever.

Millions of drinkers wish they could be in your shoes: on the brink of being able to call yourself a nondrinker. That's a wonderful achievement. Soon you will rediscover the joy of feeling healthy, having nothing to hide, having time for the people you love and the things you love to do. You're about to get a huge part of your life back.

2. BLOW AWAY THE ILLUSIONS

Remind yourself of all the illusions that made you believe that drinking gave you pleasure and support. You know and understand that alcohol does nothing for you whatsoever; it's a poison that would eventually destroy you physically and mentally. You know that alcohol doesn't relieve stress and anxiety; it causes them. Alcohol is not a social lubricant; it's a social saboteur. Alcohol doesn't give you courage; it gives you fear. Alcohol doesn't help you think; it impairs your judgment.

You've learned to see through the myths that keep people in the alcohol trap. Think about those myths and make sure you're seeing the truth. Once you've seen through a con trick, you can't be fooled by it again.

3. UNDERSTAND ADDICTION

Remind yourself that the reason you've not been able to stop drinking permanently before is not because there is something terrific about alcohol that you can't live without, nor because of some flaw in your personality. It's simply because you followed the wrong method.

The only reason you ever thought alcohol gave you some kind of pleasure or crutch was because each drink gave you a little bit of relief from the craving caused by the drink before it. You've been hooked on a drug that takes control away from you but still tricks you into thinking you're in control. Alcohol made you a slave by inducing panic at the thought of being deprived of your next drink —an addiction that is 99 percent mental and 1 percent physical. Now you know that the only way to remove that panic is to stop drinking.

4. REMOVE ALL DOUBT

If you can check the first three items on the check list, you should also be able to check item 4. Just as you wouldn't jump out of an airplane door if you weren't absolutely certain that you'd packed your parachute correctly, you should only go through the ritual of the final drink if you're in no doubt whatsoever that the decision you're taking is not only the right one; it's the *only* one.

Prepare yourself mentally for any lingering pangs that you feel after you've stopped, so that you're clear that they are just the dying cries of the Little Monster and you can enjoy them, knowing that they spell

FREEDOM!

If you have doubts about what you are about to do and can't complete the check list, there's something you haven't understood. It's essential that you go back and reread the relevant section until you do. If this applies to you, don't worry. A lot of people get to this stage and feel unsure about one aspect or another. It nearly always turns out to be just one small detail that they haven't quite grasped and all it takes for your mind to click is to go back and read it once more.

PICKING YOUR MOMENT

It's quite typical among people trying to quit drinking and other addictions to time their attempt to coincide with a certain occasion, such as a birthday or vacation. What they're effectively doing is giving themselves a deadline beyond which they're no longer allowed to drink. New Year's Day is the most commonly chosen occasion, it being a date when we "ring out the old and ring in the new." If we're looking to start afresh, free from alcohol, it seems as good a time as any, doesn't it? You might be surprised to learn that people who try to quit on New Year's Day actually have the lowest success rate.

We drink so much during the Christmas holidays that by New Year's Eve we're just about ready for a break. One last binge and then, as the clock strikes midnight, we vow that we'll give the stuff a wide berth. After a few days we're starting to feel cleansed, but the Little Monster is screaming for its fix. If we haven't killed the Big Monster, we interpret these cries as "I need a drink." Eventually the screams of the Little Monster outweigh our dwindling aversion to drink and before long we're right back in the trap.

New Year's Eve is the most extreme example, but it's typical of any special occasion used to quit. We call these "meaningless days" because they actually have no bearing whatsoever on your drinking, other than providing a deadline for you to begin your attempt to stop. Ask yourself why you need a deadline? Aren't you just saying, "I will quit, just not today. I'll let myself carry on for a while, but after that date I'll be firm with myself?" There are two problems with this:

1. You should have absolutely no desire to carry on.

2. Quitting doesn't require you to be firm with yourself. It's easy.

Meaningless days force us to quit against our will and so bring on the feeling of deprivation. When we fail, it reinforces the belief that stopping is very hard. This damaging cycle leaves drinkers spending their lives making half-hearted attempts to quit and always looking for excuses to put off "the dreaded day."

Some people choose a vacation as their time to quit because

they think it will give them a bit more time away from their usual routine. Others choose a time when there are no social events coming up where they presume they might find it difficult not to drink. These approaches might work for a while, but they leave a lingering doubt: "OK, I've coped so far, but what about when I go back to work or that big party comes around?"

With Easyway we encourage you to carry on living as normal. Go out and handle stress; throw yourself into social occasions; let your hair down, so that you can prove to yourself from the start that, even at times when you feared you would find it hard to cope without drinking, you're still happy to be free.

So when is the best time to quit?

If you saw someone you love hurting themselves repeatedly and unnecessarily, what would you say? Would you suggest they stop the next time a convenient moment arises? Or would you suggest that they stop at once?

THE IDEAL MOMENT TO STOP IS RIGHT NOW!

When you quit with Easyway, you remove all desire to drink, and so there is no point in letting yourself carry on, not for a month, not for a week, not even for a day. If you had a friend who was in an abusive relationship that was leaving her physically and mentally damaged and she told you she was thinking of walking out, what would you tell her?

DON'T WAIT FOR "THE RIGHT TIME" TO QUIT

DO IT NOW!

Living with an alcohol problem is just like living with an abusive partner. It leaves you physically battered, destroys your confidence and self-esteem, yet makes you feel perversely dependent on your abuser. The only difference is that you can walk out on drink any time you like and no one will try to stop you.

You have everything you need to quit. A much better life awaits you as soon as you do, a life free from slavery and self-loathing. It's time to rediscover your appetite for life, your energy, creativity, and libido. No more hangovers, sleepless nights, and lost days. No more lying and deceit trying to conceal your shame. No more feeling disappointed, ashamed, guilty, and weak because your latest bout of drinking has made a fool of you or taken you somewhere you really did not want to be.

You have a right to happiness. Look forward to living in the light with your head held high, enjoying open, honest relationships with the people around you, feeling in control of how you spend your time and money, and finding joy in the genuine pleasures that you enjoyed before you walked into the alcohol trap. Enjoy the return of your incredible senses—touch and smell especially.

With so much happiness to gain and so much misery to rid yourself of, what possible reason is there to wait?

SIXTH INSTRUCTION: DON'T WAIT FOR THE RIGHT TIME TO QUIT. DO IT NOW!

THE "RATIONALIZED" LIST

Go through each point and ask yourself:

• Do I understand it? • Do I agree with it? • Am I following it?

If you have any doubts, reread the relevant chapters as listed.

R	**REJOICE!**
	There's nothing to lose and everything to gain.
	Chapters 5, 14, 16
A	**ADVICE**
	Ignore it if it conflicts with Easyway.
	Chapter 9
T	**TIMING**
	Do it now!
	Chapter 17
I	**ILLUSIONS**
	Alcohol gives you neither pleasure nor a crutch.
	Chapters 2, 3, 6, 7, 10, 12
O	**ONE DRINK**
	Is all it takes to hook you again.
	Chapter 12
N	**NEVER**
	Drink or even crave a drink.
	Chapters 14, 15
A	**ADDICTIVE PERSONALITY**
	There's no such thing.
	Chapter 10
L	**LIFESTYLE**
	Rediscover genuine pleasures.
	Chapters 3, 14
I	**IMMEDIATE**
	Get back your enthusiasm for life!
	Chapters 14, 16
Z	**ZEST**
	You are not "giving up" anything.
	Chapters 3, 5, 7, 10, 12
E	**ELEPHANTS**
	Don't try not to think about drinking.
	Chapter 14
D	**DOUBT**
	Never doubt your decision to quit.
	Chapters 8, 10, 16

Remember how you felt when you started reading this book. With most drinkers we meet it's a mixture of hope and skepticism. They love the idea of being able to free themselves from their drink problem but find it hard to believe that it can really be easy. As you go through the method, however, it becomes evident that there is no effort required on your part; all you have to do is follow the instructions. It's as easy as walking from one place to another. Just keep putting one foot in front of the other and you can't fail to get there. You have now reached the end of that walk. It may have looked like a long walk at the beginning, but now you have arrived you know how easy it is.

ALL YOU HAD TO DO WAS OPEN YOUR MIND AND ALLOW YOURSELF TO SEE THE TRUE PICTURE.

Any skepticism you had at the start should now have been replaced by belief.

You have seen for yourself that the claims we made are true and so any preconceptions you had about the final drink and the withdrawal period should also have been blown away.

YOU'RE READY!

All that remains is to make sure you finish the book.

> If you're hesitating, please go through the RATIONALIZED list again or call your nearest Allen Carr's Easyway To Stop Drinking Center if you have any questions.

SUMMARY

- Make sure you're in a positive frame of mind
- Remind yourself of all the illusions that kept you in the trap
- Go over everything you understand about addiction
- If you have any lingering doubts, use the RATIONALIZED check list to identify them and reread the relevant sections

- SIXTH INSTRUCTION: DON'T WAIT FOR THE RIGHT TIME TO QUIT. DO IT NOW!

Chapter 18

THE FINAL DRINK

The final drink is the point at which you break the cycle of addiction. It's important that you observe the ritual for this reason. Once you've completed it, you are free.

Can you believe you've actually reached this point? You're about to make the final move that completes your escape from slavery to alcohol. That's an incredible achievement—literally incredible for millions of drinkers, who believe that quitting is so hard that it's beyond their capabilities. If only they knew what you know now.

You're getting your life back, rediscovering genuine pleasures, freeing yourself from slavery and torment, improving your health and wealth. In short, you're taking control of your life so you can live it the way everyone wants to live:

HAPPY AND FREE!

Quitting with Easyway is as simple as following a set of instructions, but it still requires discipline and perseverance. At any point you could have lost faith in the method and gone back to the prison, but you didn't. You kept an open mind and allowed the truth to replace the brainwashing. That takes courage. So be proud of your achievement. You've reached a position that millions of drinkers dream about: You're standing on the brink of freedom.

Remember, if you feel nervous, it's nothing to worry about. A few butterflies in the stomach are completely normal at this stage and are no threat to your chances of success. They are a sign of excitement and nothing else. When you make a parachute jump, the last-minute nerves quickly turn to exhilaration as your parachute opens and you realize that everything you've learned and prepared for is working exactly how they told you it would. You are about to feel a similar exhilaration when you finish your final drink and make a solemn vow never to drink again.

IN HER OWN WORDS: SARAH

I quit drinking with Easyway and I know I'll never touch another drink again in my life. It's opened my eyes: I can see now that I didn't even enjoy drinking, but my addiction made me neglect other important areas of my life: my children, my health, my home. I feel all the benefits that Easyway promised: I feel healthy, full of energy, and I've learned to respect myself again. The self-loathing has gone. I feel in control and it shows—I've been told by my husband that the change in my mood is amazing.

There is nothing more uplifting to behold than the utter joy of the person who has finally accepted that they don't need to drink any more. Their elation is extraordinary. One minute they're trapped in a vile, dark prison, the next they're standing in the sunlight, free of all that pain and misery, with all the joys the world has to offer available to them again. Getting free is like having a huge, dark shadow removed from your life. You no longer have any reason to worry about what you've been doing to your health, or about all the money that you've been wasting. The panic about where the next drink is coming from disappears and there's no more of that terrible self-loathing that dogs you every time the desire to drink gets the better of you again. You no longer regard yourself as weak, sordid, or pathetic. You see yourself as you really are: a wonderful human being with lots to offer and lots to enjoy from life.

As you prepare for the ritual of the final drink, remind yourself that by quitting drinking you're gaining access to all the good things in life—you're not "giving up" anything. You had no need to drink before you started and you have no need to drink now. You've analyzed the illusion of pleasure and seen that there is no genuine pleasure in drinking. You've asked how drink can possibly help in stressful situations and seen that drink provides no kind of crutch whatsoever. If you've followed and understood everything up to this point, you'll have come to the obvious conclusion:

THERE IS NO REASON TO DRINK

IN HER OWN WORDS: KATHRYN

At the age of 25 I thought life couldn't get any better. By the age of 35 I thought it couldn't get any worse. I had a good job, a lovely boyfriend, a great social life, my own apartment, I played tennis every weekend and loved it and I was proud of my health and fitness. Then my drinking got the better of me. I lost my fitness, then my boyfriend, then my job, and finally my apartment. I watched it all slip through my fingers, but with each new blow I tried to console myself with drink. I honestly thought I'd had it. I looked ahead and saw nothing but misery for the rest of my life, which I couldn't see stretching much beyond 40. To be honest, I didn't want it to. I hoped the drink would take me as soon as possible.

But now I'm 41 and I've been off the booze for two years, thanks to Easyway. It made me see I was trapped in a vicious circle and if I could only break the circle by stopping drinking it would fall apart and I would walk free. That's exactly what happened. Now I'm working again, I have a new apartment, and I've just gotten back with my old boyfriend. Life is wonderful, but the most wonderful thing of all is knowing that the drink will never take me again because I no longer feel any need for it. I used to think it was the icing on the cake, now I know the cake tastes much better without it. You won't believe how good it is to be free until you feel it for yourself.

IT'S TIME

You're ready to walk free from the alcohol trap. You'll be asked to have one final drink and then to make a solemn vow never to drink again. If you've already had what you regard as your final drink and are absolutely certain that you have no desire to drink again, you might think there's no need for this ritual. We're not about to make you go back on that final drink and have another, but we will ask you to make the vow.

This is one of the most important decisions you'll ever make. You're freeing yourself from slavery and achieving something fantastic, something all drinkers would love to achieve and something that everybody, drinkers and nondrinkers alike, will admire you for. You're about to go right up in the estimation of one person in particular: yourself. This is an ecstatic moment and it deserves to be marked with some ceremony.

But the most important purpose of the ritual is to draw a clear line between where your drinking ends and your new freedom begins. The thing that makes quitting hard with other methods is not the physical aggravation of withdrawal; it's the lack of certainty, the eternal waiting to become a nondrinker. With Easyway you get certainty straightaway. There is nothing to wait for. You become a nondrinker the moment you finish your final drink and you confirm your commitment to become a nondrinker when you make your vow. It's important to know when that moment is, to be able to make that vow with a feeling of real intent, to visualize your triumph over the two monsters and be able to say, "Yes! I'm a nondrinker now. I'm FREE!"

If you haven't already stopped drinking, pour your final drink now. If you have, think about that drink and follow the ritual from here.

Make yourself comfortable, relax, and check your state of mind. It's essential that you're completely reconciled with the notion of never drinking again. You must be absolutely clear that drinking gives you no pleasure or crutch whatsoever and that you are not making any sort of sacrifice. Let's recap over the things that may cause you to doubt your decision:

1. The belief that you're making a genuine sacrifice.

Does it bother you unduly that you might never eat caviar again in your life? Caviar is considered a genuine delicacy, yet you could easily live without caviar for the rest of your life and not feel deprived. Drinking gives no genuine pleasure or crutch whatsoever. The fact that it appeared to was just a subtle illusion.

THERE IS ABSOLUTELY NOTHING TO GIVE UP

2. Thebeliefthatit'spossibletohavetheoccasionaldrinkwithout getting hooked.

Why would you want to? Regardless of what casual drinkers want you to think, they are just as addicted as heavy drinkers, but they feel more deprived.

*THERE IS ONLY ONE WAY TO FEEL LIKE A
NONDRINKER AND THAT IS TO NOT DRINK*

*THE ONLY ESSENTIAL IN ORDER TO BE A
NONDRINKER FOR LIFE IS NEVER TO DRINK*

*IN ORDER TO BE A HAPPY NONDRINKER FOR LIFE, IT
IS ESSENTIAL NEVER TO DESIRE TO DRINK*

If you have a desire to have just one drink, you will have a desire to drink another and another. Be absolutely clear: It has to be all or nothing.

3. The belief that you're a confirmed drinker, or have an addictive personality, or are in some way different from all other people.

You got hooked because you took an addictive drug. The traits that are common to addicts are caused by the addiction; they don't cause it. Anyone can fall for the alcohol trap.

*A DRINK PROBLEM IS CAUSED BY THE DRINK,
NOT THE DRINKER*

4.   Other drinkers.

All drinkers lie in order to justify their illogical behavior, but you've seen through the illusions and you know the truth. Remember, they're the ones who are losing out, not you.

DRINKERS LIE BECAUSE THEY FEEL STUPID

You've reached this exciting point in the method without pain or hardship. You've proven that it's ridiculously easy to stop drinking provided you follow all the instructions. You're stopping because you're sick of being a slave to alcohol, so make sure your mindset is not "I must never drink again", but "This is great! I don't ever need to waste my time and money on making myself miserable again.

I'M WALKING FREE!"

THE VOW AND THE FINAL DRINK

As you drink your final drink—or reconjure your final drink in your mind—focus on how it smells and the taste it leaves in your mouth.

Ask yourself if the misery you've suffered was worth it. Be aware that any feeling of pleasure is merely relief at the Little Monster being quietened for a while.

I WOULD NOW LIKE YOU TO CONSUME YOUR FINAL DRINK.

REJOICE! YOU ARE NOW FREE!

Visualize that monster and make a solemn vow to destroy it once and for all. Say out loud,

I VOW THAT I WILL NEVER DRINK AGAIN BECAUSE I HAVE NO DESIRE TO DRINK.

I VOW THAT I AM COMMITTED TO FREEING MYSELF FROM ALCOHOL AND BECOMING A HAPPY NONDRINKER FOR THE REST OF MY LIFE.

I VOW THAT I HAVE HAD MY FINAL DRINK.

I AM FREE!

The ritual ends here. The vow marks the breaking of the cycle of addiction, in which each fix created the need or desire for the next. By breaking the cycle you've removed the cause of the desire.

You've put down a marker in your mind. This is the moment when you find yourself on the outside of the prison. Think back to the misery and suffering that alcohol was causing you. Now that's all in the past. Visualize the Little Monster and how it has wound you round its little finger all this time. Imagine it laughing at you.

Now it's time for revenge. No more slavery! No more misery! Cut off its lifeline and destroy that evil tyrant once and for all.

FREEDOM STARTS HERE

Now you can move on. There is no need to wait for a response. Embrace this moment with a feeling of elation. You've jumped, your parachute is open, you're floating blissfully to the ground, and all the genuine pleasures that the world has to offer are laid out before your eyes.

Rejoice in your victory. You've earned it, not through hard graft and willpower but through courage, common sense, and the ability to open your mind. These are traits you've always possessed—you just needed to be shown how to apply them.

This is one of the greatest achievements of your life, if not the greatest. It's important that it sticks in your mind. At the moment you're fired up with powerful reasons to stop, but in a few days, as you enjoy your newfound freedom, your resolution will fade. As the days, weeks, and years slip by, your memory of how drinking made you feel will dim. So fix how you feel at this moment in your mind while it's still vivid, so that even if your memory of the details should fade, your resolution never to drink again will not.

If you're prepared for a challenge, it doesn't faze you as it would if it took you by surprise. You can easily guard against any moments of doubt in future simply by knowing that they will arise. Use this moment to strengthen your foundations and you will be well prepared to handle any future challenges to your resolution to live the rest of your life as a happy nondrinker.

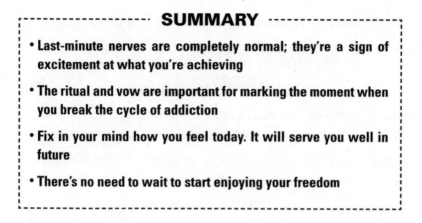

------------------------------ **SUMMARY** -------------------------------

- Last-minute nerves are completely normal; they're a sign of excitement at what you're achieving

- The ritual and vow are important for marking the moment when you break the cycle of addiction

- Fix in your mind how you feel today. It will serve you well in future

- There's no need to wait to start enjoying your freedom

Chapter 19

ENJOYING YOUR
NEW LIFE

IN THIS CHAPTER
- *THE FIRST FEW DAYS*
- *ALL YOU HAVE GAINED* - *COPING WITH BAD DAYS*
- *STAYING FREE FOREVER*

You've done it! You're now a nondrinker and will remain so provided you never doubt your decision and never drink again.

Congratulations! You're ready to start enjoying life as a happy nondrinker. Instead of chasing an unknown pleasure and striving in vain to rid yourself of the restless torture of addiction, you're going to rediscover the genuine pleasures of life and feel the contentment that a nondrinker feels all the time.

For the first few days after your final drink you may detect the cries of the Little Monster as it goes through its death throes. This is nothing to worry about, so don't try to push it from your mind, Recognize the cries and rejoice in what they signify—the death of the monster that has held you enslaved for all this time.

As a drinker you felt compelled to feed the Little Monster. Now you're free, you don't have to do anything. That's the method for killing the Little Monster:

DO NOTHING!

This vile parasite inside you is dying and very soon you will be rid of it altogether.

That's the beautiful secret to killing the Little Monster. In fact, it's not a secret at all; it's just that most drinkers are never told that this is the solution to their problem. They think they have to go on feeding the Little Monster and the only way to resist the temptation is by applying all their willpower.

When the Little Monster cries out, do nothing. You used to be its slave, running about trying to find alcohol to satisfy its demands. Now you don't need to. It's like being nagged to do something you don't want to do and making your mind up to sit where you are and not lift a finger. It's FABULOUS!

You don't have to blot out the nagging and pretend it's not happening. You can listen to it all you like—enjoy it. The nagging becomes a source of amusement. Let it nag itself out. It's its problem, not yours.

The Little Monster knows it has a problem and will do everything it can to make you help it out. But why should you? This is a tyrant that has held you captive for too long and now it's your turn for revenge. The more it grumbles, the more you know you've won. Rejoice in your victory.

Drinkers who quit with the willpower method are never told that the death throes are a sign that they've won, so they see them as evidence of what they always feared: that quitting will be hard.

Rather than rejoicing, they respond in negative ways: They

feel irritable, restless, angry, insecure, disorientated, or lethargic. They allow these negative feelings to make them think they might be better off drinking again, forgetting that they already suffered from these feelings when they were drinking. They're the same feelings that they always interpreted as "I need a drink".

From a physical perspective, living with the death throes is no harder than living with a mild cold for a few days. They only become a problem if you start to worry about them or interpret them as a need or desire to drink. Many people don't even feel them after they quit, but if you do, just picture a Little Monster searching around the desert for a drink and you having control of the water supply. All you have to do is keep the tap turned off. It's as easy as that.

You should have your mindset prepared so that you are ready with the right response.

Instead of thinking, "I need a drink but I'm not allowed one", think, "This is the Little Monster demanding its fix. This is what drinkers suffer throughout their drinking lives. Nondrinkers don't suffer this feeling. Isn't it great! I'm a nondrinker and so I'll soon be free of it forever."

Focus on the physical sensation and ask yourself if there is really any discomfort. If there is, remind yourself that the only reason you're feeling any discomfort at all is not because you've stopped drinking but because you started in the first place. Be clear that having another drink would not relieve the discomfort; on the contrary, it would ensure that you suffered it for the rest of your life.

YOUR NEW LIFE STARTS HERE

You become a nondrinker the moment you finish your final drink, so start getting on with the rest of your life and enjoying the many pleasures it has to offer straightaway. The Little Monster will die soon enough without you having to do anything about it.

When you were still drinking you might have found it hard to envisage what we meant by "getting on with the rest of your life". You'd lost sight of the genuine pleasures, and so the thought of having the freedom to pursue anything you wanted may have rung hollow. When you're obsessed with where your next drink is coming from, everything else in life pales into insignificance.

As soon as you come off the booze, you begin to rediscover the genuine joys of life: reading books, getting out and about, watching entertainment, socializing, exercise, sex… It's one of the best things about becoming a nondrinker. As drinkers we don't realize it's our alcohol addiction that's killed our interest and dulled our sensitivity in these pleasures and we assume it's just part of the process of getting old and jaded. Becoming a nondrinker is like becoming young again. When you're free from alcohol, it's easy to find pleasure in so many things.

You'll find that situations you've come to regard as boring or even irritating become enjoyable again: gentle pleasures like spending time with your loved ones, going for walks, seeing friends. Work will become more enjoyable too, as you find your performance improves and you're better able to concentrate, think creatively, and handle stress.

You'll also become more assertive about the things you *don't* like. Most drinkers spend time going to boring functions that give them no pleasure at all and get stuck into the drink in the belief that it will help them relax and have fun. They regard it as their weakness that they struggle to enjoy these occasions. When you stop drinking you quickly come to see that it's not a weakness on your part that these occasions seem boring—the truth is they *are* boring.

Instead of trying to change yourself in order to enjoy boring occasions, as a nondrinker you're able to make the more sensible decision and stop going to them, or, if you're obliged to go, make your excuses and leave at the first opportunity. When you cut alcohol out of your life, you regain the ability to see things as they really are and make better decisions about how you run your life.

BACK IN TRIM

There are a lot of empty calories in alcoholic drinks and this, coupled with the debilitating effect that alcohol addiction has on your energy levels, plus the tendency to eat so-called convenience food, leads many drinkers to compound their drink problem with a weight problem. Becoming a nondrinker makes it so much easier for you to shed excess pounds and get physically fit.

The biggest factor in controlling your weight is eating the correct foods. The sort of junk food that you turn to when drinking has made you feel too lethargic to cook or make healthy choices. Junk food is high in calories and low in nutrients, so it takes more of it to satisfy your hunger. The empty feeling of the Little Monster crying out for alcohol can feel very similar to hunger so, just as drinkers often try to satisfy their hunger by drinking, they also try to satisfy their alcohol craving by eating.

Just as alcohol and junk food tend to go hand in hand, when you stop drinking you quickly rediscover the pleasure of eating fresh, healthy food that quickly satisfies your hunger and makes you feel good. If you want to learn more about gaining control of your weight through healthy eating, read Allen Carr's *Lose Weight Now* or *The Easy Way for Women to Lose Weight*.

Exercise is another of the genuine pleasures in life that you rediscover when you stop drinking. That said, we don't advocate exercising to lose weight for the simple reason that, like the willpower method, it feels like a hardship and it doesn't work. The more you exercise, the more calories you burn, and so the more you need to eat. It's a balance that's designed by nature to ensure you maintain a constant weight. Eat only when you're hungry, eat the food that gives you the nutrients you need and nothing more, and you will achieve your ideal weight.

The obsession with exercising to lose excess weight is the direct result of eating the wrong types of food. You only have to look at the market for second-hand exercise bikes, rowing machines, and all the other instruments of torture that people splash out on in the hope that they will help them lose weight to see that they don't work. This sort of exercise demands willpower. It may give you a sense of pride to begin with, but it quickly feels like penance. It also makes you hungry. So what do you do? Reward yourself with a cake, chocolate bar, or some other piece of junk food that defeats the object of exercising in the first place.

Exercise for pleasure, on the other hand, is a wonderful thing and something you will feel more and more inclined to take up as your weight drops and your energy level rises. It could be anything from walking in the countryside to a competitive sport —the most important thing is that you do it for pleasure. If you've become unfit, take it easy to begin with and step it up gradually as your fitness improves. Incorporating opportunities to move your body in the normal routine of your life is wonderful. Walk a while rather than take the car or bus. Use the stairs, not the elevator. It's wonderful to move your body in these seemingly effortless ways.

Whatever exercise you take up, you'll find it gives you a greater appetite. As long as you continue to eat the right foods and eat only when hungry, you won't put on weight. This is the virtuous circle that nature designed for all creatures, to ensure they remain healthy and strong throughout their natural lives.

The cycle of healthy eating and exercise is not something you have to work at. You'll feel it working for you right from the start. Your weight will go down because you're no longer overloading your body with unwanted junk. You'll feel healthier and your energy levels will rise. You won't have to force yourself to take exercise; you will be champing at the bit to get out there. Just make sure that the exercise is enjoyable.

In addition to feeling stronger, slimmer, and more energetic, you'll feel more lighthearted too. It's been proven that exercise releases happy hormones, giving you a more positive perspective on life and boosting your self-esteem. You'll feel more attractive, which in turn feeds back into your positivity. Just by taking drink out of your diet, you set in motion a positive cycle of contentment that continues to roll for life.

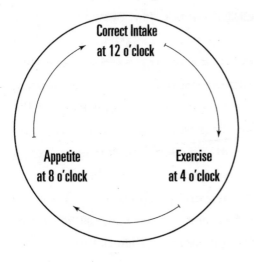

Each phase in the cycle causes the next. It is the same perfect balance that makes exercising to lose weight futile, but by getting the intake right you can turn it to your advantage—a self-perpetuating process of pleasure.

PREPARE FOR TRICKY TIMES

In a few months you'll find it hard to believe that you once felt any need to drink alcohol, let alone how much it controlled you. You'll feel completely in control and you'll lose your fear of getting hooked again. This will be a danger period, so prepare yourself now.

You could have moments when you're on a high, surrounded by drinkers, or you might suffer a trauma of some kind and your guard will be down. Never forget:

THERE'S NO SUCH THING AS JUST ONE DRINK

If you have one drink, it will inevitably lead to another and another. Be aware now that these situations could arise and make it part of your commitment to quitting that, if and when they come, you'll be ready for them and there's no way that you'll be fooled into having a drink.

Prepare too for days when it's hard to see the joy in life. Everybody, drinker or nondrinker, has bad days when everything that can go wrong does go wrong. It has nothing to do with the fact that you've stopped drinking. In fact, when you stop drinking you find the bad days don't come around so frequently, and when they do, you feel better equipped to cope with them.

Nevertheless, you might well find that when bad days come around the thought of drinking enters your mind. Don't worry about it or try to push the thought out of your mind. Just recognize that it's a remnant from the days when you responded to every setback by drinking. It doesn't mean you're still vulnerable to the trap; it just means you're still adjusting to your newfound freedom. Remember the mindset: Instead of thinking, "I mustn't drink," or "I thought I'd overcome this addiction," think, "Great! I don't have to drink any more. I'm free!" The thought will pass very quickly and the positivity will return.

You've achieved something fantastic. It's essential that you never undervalue that achievement, nor doubt or question your decision to stop. Never make the mistake that people on the willpower method make of craving another drink. If you do, you will put yourself in the same impossible position as them: miserable if you don't, even more miserable if you do. The final instruction is one that you have already decided for yourself:

SEVENTH INSTRUCTION: NEVER EVER DRINK AGAIN!

SUMMARY

- Enjoy the death throes of the Little Monster
- Don't wait to start enjoying life as a nondrinker
- Take exercise for pleasure, not as a means to lose weight
- Be prepared for bad days—you'll handle them better as a nondrinker
- SEVENTH INSTRUCTION: NEVER EVER DRINK ALCOHOL AGAIN!

Chapter 20

USEFUL REMINDERS

Here's a summary of the key points that we've discussed, together with a reminder of the instructions. You might find it useful to remind yourself of these points from time to time.

- **Don't wait for anything. You're already a nondrinker from the moment you finish your final drink. You've cut off the supply to the Little Monster and unlocked the door of your prison.**

- **Accept that there will always be good days and bad days. Because you will be stronger both physically and mentally within no time at all, you'll enjoy the good times more and handle the bad times better.**

- **Be aware that a very important change is happening in your life. Like all major changes, it can take time for your mind and body to adjust. Don't worry if you feel different or disorientated for a few days. Just accept it as part of your liberation.**

- **Remember you've stopped drinking; you haven't stopped living. You can start enjoying life to the full straightaway.**

- **There's no need to avoid other drinkers. Go out and enjoy social** occasions and show yourself you can handle them right from the start.

• Don't envy drinkers. When you're with them, remind yourself you're not being deprived; they are. They will be envying you because they wish they could be free.

• Never doubt your decision to stop—you know it's the right one. Never mope about not drinking. If you do, you'll put yourself in an impossible position: You will be miserable if you don't and even more miserable if you do.

• Make sure right from the start that if the thought of "just one drink" enters your mind, you think, "YIPPEE! I'm a nondrinker." The thought will pass very quickly from your brain and it will learn not to think it again.

• Don't try not to think about drinking. It's impossible to make your brain not think about something. You will make yourself frustrated and miserable. It's easy to think about drinking without feeling miserable: Instead of thinking, "I mustn't drink," or "When will the craving stop?" think, "Great! I'm a nondrinker. Yippee! I'm free!"

THE INSTRUCTIONS

1. FOLLOW ALL THE INSTRUCTIONS IN ORDER

2. KEEP AN OPEN MIND

3. START WITH A FEELING OF ELATION

4. NEVER DOUBT YOUR DECISION TO QUIT

5. IGNOREALLADVICEANDINFLUENCESTHATCONFLICT WITH EASYWAY

6. DON'TWAITFORTHERIGHTTIMETOQUIT.DOITNOW!

7. ONCE YOU'VE STOPPED, NEVER DRINK AGAIN!

LIST OF ALLEN CARR'S EASYWAY CENTERS

The following list indicates the countries where Allen Carr's Easyway To Stop Smoking Centers are currently operational.

Check www.allencarr.com for latest additions to this list.

The success rate at the centers, based on the three-month, money-back guarantee, is over 90 percent.

Selected centers also offer sessions that deal with alcohol, other drugs, and weight issues. Please check with your nearest center, listed below, for details.

Allen Carr's Easyway guarantee that you will find it easy to stop at the centers or your money back.

JOIN US!

Allen Carr's Easyway Centers have spread throughout the world with incredible speed and success. Our global franchise network now covers more than 150 cities in over 45 countries. This amazing growth has been achieved entirely organically. Former addicts, just like you, were so impressed by the ease with which they stopped that they felt inspired to contact us to see how they could bring the method to their region.

If you feel the same, contact us for details on how to become an Allen Carr's Easyway To Stop Smoking or an Allen Carr's Easyway To Stop Drinking franchisee.

Email us at: **join-us@allencarr.com** including your full name, postal address, and region of interest.

SUPPORT US!

No, don't send us money!

You have achieved something really marvellous. Every time we hear of someone escaping from the sinking ship, we get a feeling of enormous satisfaction.

It would give us great pleasure to hear that you have freed yourself from the slavery of addiction so please visit the following web page where you can tell us of your success, inspire others to follow in your footsteps and hear about ways you can help to spread the word.

www.allencarr.com/fanzone

You can "like" our facebook page here
www.facebook.com/AllenCarr

Together, we can help further Allen Carr's mission: to cure the world of addiction.

ALLEN CARR'S EASYWAY CENTERS

LONDON CLINIC AND WORLDWIDE HEAD OFFICE

Park House, 14 Pepys Road, Raynes Park, London SW20 8NH

Tel: +44 (0)20 8944 7761

Fax: +44 (0)20 8944 8619

Email: mail@allencarr.com

Website: www.allencarr.com

Therapists: John Dicey, Colleen Dwyer, Crispin Hay, Emma Hudson, Rob Fielding, Sam Kelser, Rob Groves, Debbie Brewer-West, Mark Keen, Duncan Bhaskaran-Brown, Mark Newman, Gerry Williams (Alcohol), Monique Douglas (Weight)

WORLDWIDE PRESS OFFICE

Tel: +44 (0)7970 88 44 52

Contact: John Dicey

Tel: +44 (0)7970 88 44 52

Email: media@allencarr.com

NORTH AMERICAN CENTERS

U.S.A.

Sessions held throughout the USA

Tel: +1 855 440 3777

Email: support@usa.allencarr.com

Website: www.allencarr.com

New York

Tel: +1 855 440 3777

Therapists: Natalie Clays and Team

Email: support@usa.allencarr.com

Website: www.allencarr.com

Los Angeles

Tel: +1 855 440 3777

Therapists: Natalie Clays and Team

Email: support@usa.allencarr.com

Website: www.allencarr.com

Milwaukee (and South Wisconsin)

Tel: +1 262 770 1260

Therapist: Wayne Spaulding

Email: wayne@easywaywisconsin.com

Website: www.allencarr.com

CANADA

Tel: +1 855 440 3777

Therapist: Natalie Clays

Email: natalie@ca.allencarr.com

Website: www.allencarr.com

U.K. CENTERS

Birmingham
Tel & Fax: 0800 389 2115
Therapists: John Dicey, Colleen
Dwyer, Crispin Hay, Emma Hudson,
Rob Fielding, Sam Kelser, Rob Groves,
Debbie Brewer-West, Mark Keen,
Duncan Bhaskaran-Brown, Mark
Newman
Email: mail@allencarr.com
Website: www.allencarr.com

Bournemouth
Tel: 0800 389 2115
Therapists: John Dicey, Colleen
Dwyer, Crispin Hay, Emma Hudson,
Rob Fielding, Sam Kelser, Rob Groves,
Debbie Brewer-West, Mark Keen,
Duncan Bhaskaran-Brown, Mark
Newman
Email: mail@allencarr.com
Website: www.allencarr.com

Brentwood
Tel: 0800 389 2115
Therapists: John Dicey, Colleen
Dwyer, Crispin Hay, Emma Hudson,
Rob Fielding, Sam Kelser, Rob Groves,
Debbie Brewer-West, Mark Keen,
Duncan Bhaskaran-Brown, Mark
Newman
Email: mail@allencarr.com
Website: www.allencarr.com

Brighton
Tel: 0800 389 2115
Therapists: John Dicey, Colleen
Dwyer, Crispin Hay, Emma Hudson,
Rob Fielding, Sam Kelser, Rob Groves,
Debbie Brewer-West, Mark Keen,
Duncan Bhaskaran-Brown, Mark
Newman
Email: mail@allencarr.com
Website: www.allencarr.com

Bristol
Tel: 0800 389 2115
Therapists: John Dicey, Colleen
Dwyer, Crispin Hay, Emma Hudson,
Rob Fielding, Sam Kelser, Rob Groves,
Debbie Brewer-West, Mark Keen,
Duncan Bhaskaran-Brown, Mark
Newman
Email: mail@allencarr.com
Website: www.allencarr.com

Cambridge
Tel: 0800 389 2115
Therapists: John Dicey, Colleen
Dwyer, Crispin Hay, Emma Hudson,
Rob Fielding, Sam Kelser, Rob Groves,
Debbie Brewer-West, Mark Keen,
Duncan Bhaskaran-Brown, Mark
Newman
Email: mail@allencarr.com
Website: www.allencarr.com

Coventry
Tel: 0800 321 3007
Therapist: Rob Fielding
Email: info@easywaymidlands.co.uk
Website: www.allencarr.com

Cumbria
Tel: 0800 389 2115
Therapists: John Dicey, Colleen
Dwyer, Crispin Hay, Emma Hudson,
Rob Fielding, Sam Kelser, Rob Groves,
Debbie Brewer-West, Mark Keen,
Duncan Bhaskaran-Brown, Mark
Newman
Email: mail@allencarr.com
Website: www.allencarr.com

Derby
Tel: 0800 389 2115
Therapists: John Dicey, Colleen
Dwyer, Crispin Hay, Emma Hudson,
Rob Fielding, Sam Kelser, Rob Groves,
Debbie Brewer-West, Mark Keen,
Duncan Bhaskaran-Brown, Mark
Newman
Email: mail@allencarr.com
Website: www.allencarr.com

Guernsey
Tel: 0800 077 6187
Therapist: Mark Keen
Email: mark@easywaymanchester.co.uk
Website: www.allencarr.com

Isle of Man
Tel: 0800 077 6187
Therapist: Mark Keen
Email: mark@easywaymanchester.co.uk
Website: www.allencarr.com

Jersey
Tel: 0800 077 6187
Therapist: Mark Keen
Email: mark@easywaymanchester.co.uk
Website: www.allencarr.com

Kent
Tel: 0800 389 2115
Therapists: John Dicey, Colleen
Dwyer, Crispin Hay, Emma Hudson,
Rob Fielding, Sam Kelser, Rob Groves,
Debbie Brewer-West, Mark Keen,
Duncan Bhaskaran-Brown, Mark
Newman
Email: mail@allencarr.com
Website: www.allencarr.com

Lancashire
Tel: 0800 389 2115
Therapists: John Dicey, Colleen
Dwyer, Crispin Hay, Emma Hudson,
Rob Fielding, Sam Kelser, Rob Groves,
Debbie Brewer-West, Mark Keen,
Duncan Bhaskaran-Brown, Mark
Newman
Email: mail@allencarr.com
Website: www.allencarr.com

Leeds
Tel: 0800 077 6187
Therapist: Mark Keen
Email: mark@easywaymanchester.co.uk
Website: www.allencarr.com

Leicester
Tel: 0800 321 3007
Therapist: Rob Fielding
Email: info@easywaymidlands.co.uk
Website: www.allencarr.com

Lincoln
Tel: 0800 321 3007
Therapist: Rob Fielding
Email: info@easywaymidlands.co.uk
Website: www.allencarr.com

Liverpool
Tel: 0800 389 2115
Therapists: John Dicey, Colleen
Dwyer, Crispin Hay, Emma Hudson,
Rob Fielding, Sam Kelser, Rob Groves,
Debbie Brewer-West, Mark Keen,
Duncan Bhaskaran-Brown, Mark
Newman
Email: mail@allencarr.com
Website: www.allencarr.com

Manchester
Tel: 0800 077 6187
Therapist: Mark Keen
Email: mark@easywaymanchester.co.uk
Website: www.allencarr.com

Milton Keynes
Tel: 0800 389 2115
Therapists: John Dicey, Colleen
Dwyer, Crispin Hay, Emma Hudson,
Rob Fielding, Sam Kelser, Rob Groves,
Debbie Brewer-West, Mark Keen,
Duncan Bhaskaran-Brown, Mark
Newman
Email: mail@allencarr.com
Website: www.allencarr.com

Newcastle/North East
Tel: 0800 389 2115
Therapists: John Dicey, Colleen
Dwyer, Crispin Hay, Emma Hudson,
Rob Fielding, Sam Kelser, Rob Groves,
Debbie Brewer-West, Mark Keen,
Duncan Bhaskaran-Brown, Mark
Newman
Email: mail@allencarr.com
Website: www.allencarr.com

Nottingham
Tel: 0800 389 2115
Therapists: John Dicey, Colleen
Dwyer, Crispin Hay, Emma Hudson,
Rob Fielding, Sam Kelser, Rob Groves,
Debbie Brewer-West, Mark Keen,

Duncan Bhaskaran-Brown, Mark
Newman
Email: mail@allencarr.com
Website: www.allencarr.com

Oxford
Tel: 0800 389 2115
Therapists: John Dicey, Colleen
Dwyer, Crispin Hay, Emma Hudson,
Rob Fielding, Sam Kelser, Rob Groves,
Debbie Brewer-West, Mark Keen,
Duncan Bhaskaran-Brown, Mark
Newman
Email: mail@allencarr.com
Website: www.allencarr.com

Reading
Tel: 0800 389 2115
Therapists: John Dicey, Colleen
Dwyer, Crispin Hay, Emma Hudson,
Rob Fielding, Sam Kelser, Rob Groves,
Debbie Brewer-West, Mark Keen,
Duncan Bhaskaran-Brown, Mark
Newman
Email: mail@allencarr.com
Website: www.allencarr.com

SCOTLAND
Glasgow and Edinburgh
Tel: +44 (0)131 449 7858
Therapists: Paul Melvin and Jim
McCreadie
Email: info@easywayscotland.co.uk
Website: www.allencarr.com

Southampton
Tel: 0800 389 2115
Therapists: John Dicey, Colleen
Dwyer, Crispin Hay, Emma Hudson,
Rob Fielding, Sam Kelser, Rob Groves,
Debbie Brewer-West, Mark Keen,
Duncan Bhaskaran-Brown, Mark
Newman
Email: mail@allencarr.com
Website: www.allencarr.com

Southport
Tel: 0800 389 2115
Therapist:s John Dicey, Colleen

Dwyer, Crispin Hay, Emma Hudson,
Rob Fielding, Sam Kelser, Rob Groves,
Debbie Brewer-West, Mark Keen,
Duncan Bhaskaran-Brown, Mark
Newman
Email: mail@allencarr.com
Website: www.allencarr.com

Staines/Heathrow
Tel: 0800 389 2115
Therapists: John Dicey, Colleen
Dwyer, Crispin Hay, Emma Hudson,
Rob Fielding, Sam Kelser, Rob Groves,
Debbie Brewer-West, Mark Keen,
Duncan Bhaskaran-Brown, Mark
Newman
Email: mail@allencarr.com
Website: www.allencarr.com

Stevenage
Tel: 0800 389 2115
Therapists: John Dicey, Colleen
Dwyer, Crispin Hay, Emma Hudson,
Rob Fielding, Sam Kelser, Rob Groves,
Debbie Brewer-West, Mark Keen,
Duncan Bhaskaran-Brown, Mark
Newman
Email: mail@allencarr.com
Website: www.allencarr.com

Stoke
Tel: 0800 389 2115
Therapists: John Dicey, Colleen
Dwyer, Crispin Hay, Emma Hudson,
Rob Fielding, Sam Kelser, Rob Groves,
Debbie Brewer-West, Mark Keen,
Duncan Bhaskaran-Brown, Mark
Newman
Email: mail@allencarr.com
Website: www.allencarr.com

Surrey
Park House, 14 Pepys Road, Raynes
Park, London SW20 8NH
Tel: +44 (0)20 8944 7761
Fax: +44 (0)20 8944 8619
Therapists: John Dicey, Colleen
Dwyer, Crispin Hay, Emma Hudson,
Rob Fielding, Sam Kelser, Rob Groves,

Debbie Brewer-West, Mark Keen,
Duncan Bhaskaran-Brown, Mark
Newman, Gerry Williams (Alcohol),
Monique Douglas (Weight)
Email: mail@allencarr.com
Website: www.allencarr.com

Watford
Tel: 0800 389 2115
Therapists: John Dicey, Colleen
Dwyer, Crispin Hay, Emma Hudson,
Rob Fielding, Sam Kelser, Rob Groves,
Debbie Brewer-West, Mark Keen,
Duncan Bhaskaran-Brown, Mark
Newman
Email: mail@allencarr.com
Website: www.allencarr.com

Worcester
Tel: 0800 321 3007
Therapist: Rob Fielding
Email: info@easywaymidlands.co.uk
Website: www.allencarr.com

WORLDWIDE CENTERS

AUSTRALIA
ACT, NSW, NT, QLD, VIC
Tel: 1300 848 028
Therapists: Natalie Clays and Team
Email: natalie@allencarr.com.au
Website: www.allencarr.com

South Australia
Tel: 1300 848 028
Therapist: Jaime Reed
Email: sa@allencarr.com.au
Website: www.allencarr.com

Western Australia
Tel: 1300 848 028
Therapist: Natalie Clays and Team
Email: natalie@allencarr.com.au
Website: www.allencarr.com

AUSTRIA
Sessions held throughout Austria
Freephone: 0800RAUCHEN (0800
7282436)
Tel: +43 (0)3512 44755
Therapists: Erich Kellermann and Team
Email: info@allen-carr.at
Website: www.allencarr.com

BELGIUM
Brussels
Tel: +32 (0)2 808 19 65
Therapist: Paula Rooduijn
Email: info@allencarr.be
Website: www.allencarr.com

BRAZIL
Therapist: Lilian Brunstein
Email: contato@easywayonline.com.br
Website: www.allencarr.com

BULGARIA
Tel: 0800 14104 / +359 899 88 99 07
Therapist: Rumyana Kostadinova
Email: rk@nepushaveche.com
Website: www.allencarr.com

CANADA
Tel: +1 855 440 3777
Therapist: Natalie Clays
Email: natalie@ca.allencarr.com
Website: www.allencarr.com

CHILE
Tel: +56 2 4744587
Therapist: Claudia Sarmiento
Email: contacto@allencarr.cl
Website: www.allencarr.com

CYPRUS
Tel: +357 25770611
Therapist: Andreas Damianou
Email: info@allencarr.com.cy
Website: www.allencarr.com

DENMARK
Sessions held throughout Denmark
Tel: +45 70267711
Therapist: Mette Fønss
Email: mette@easyway.dk
Website: www.allencarr.com

ESTONIA
Tel: +372 733 0044
Therapist: Henry Jakobson
Email: info@allencarr.ee
Website: www.allencarr.com

FINLAND
Tel: +358-(0)45 3544099
Therapist: Janne Ström
Email: info@allencarr.fi
Website: www.allencarr.com

FRANCE
Sessions held throughout France
Freephone: 0800 386387
Tel: +33 (4)91 33 54 55
Therapists: Erick Serre and Team
Email: info@allencarr.fr
Website: www.allencarr.com

GERMANY
Sessions held throughout Germany
Freephone: 08000RAUCHEN (0800 07282436)
Tel: +49 (0) 8031 90190-0
Therapists: Erich Kellermann and Team
Email: info@allen-carr.de
Website: www.allencarr.com

GREECE
Sessions held throughout Greece
Tel: +30 210 5224087
Therapist: Panos Tzouras
Email: panos@allencarr.gr
Website: www.allencarr.com

GUATEMALA
Tel: +502 2362 0000
Therapist: Michelle Binford
Email: info@dejadefumarfacil.com
Website: www.allencarr.com

HONG KONG
Email: info@easywayhongkong.com
Website: www.allencarr.com

HUNGARY
Sessions held in Budapest and 12 other cities across Hungary
Tel: 06 80 624 426 (freephone) or +36 20 580 9244
Therapist: Gábor Szász
Email: szasz.gabor@allencarr.hu
Website: www.allencarr.com

INDIA
Bangalore and Chennai
Tel: +91 (0)80 4154 0624
Therapist: Suresh Shottam
Email: info@easywaytostopsmoking.co.in
Website: www.allencarr.com

IRAN
Please check website for details
Tehran and Mashhad
Website: www.allencarr.com

ISRAEL
Sessions held throughout Israel
Tel: +972 (0)3 6212525
Therapists: Orit Rozen and Team
Email: info@allencarr.co.il
Website: www.allencarr.com

ITALY
Sessions held throughout Italy
Tel/Fax: +39 (0)2 7060 2438
Therapists: Francesca Cesati and Team
Email: info@easywayitalia.com
Website: www.allencarr.com

JAPAN
Sessions held throughout Japan
www.allencarr.com

LEBANON
Tel: +961 1 791 5565
Therapist: Sadek El-Assaad
Email: info@AllenCarrEasyWay.me
Website: www.allencarr.com

MAURITIUS
Tel: +230 5727 5103
Therapist: Heidi Hoareau
Email: info@allencarr.mu
Website: www.allencarr.com

MEXICO
Sessions held throughout Mexico
Tel: +52 55 2623 0631
Therapists: Jorge Davo and Team
Email: info@allencarr-mexico.com
Website: www.allencarr.com

NETHERLANDS
Sessions held throughout the
Netherlands
Allen Carr's Easyway 'stoppen met roken'
Tel: +31 53 478 43 62/
+31 900 786 77 37
Email: info@allencarr.nl
Website: www.allencarr.com

NEW ZEALAND
North Island – Auckland
Tel: +64 (0) 0800 848 028
Therapists: Natalie Clays and Team
Email: natalie@allencarr.co.nz
Website: www.allencarr.com

South Island – Wellington and Christchurch
Tel: +64 (0) 0800 848 028
Therapists: Natalie Clays and Team
Email: natalie@allencarr.co.nz

NORWAY
Therapist: Laila Thorsen
Please check website for details
Website: www.allencarr.com

PERU
Lima
Tel: +511 637 7310
Therapist: Luis Loranca
Email: lloranca@dejardefumaraltoque.com
Website: www.allencarr.com

POLAND
Sessions held throughout Poland
Tel: +48 (0)22 621 36 11
Therapist: Michael Spyrka
Email: info@allen-carr.pl
Website: www.allencarr.com

POLAND – Alcohol seminars
Please check website for details
Tel: +48 71 307 32 37
Therapist: Maciej Kramarz
Email: mk@allecarr.com.pl
Website: www.allencarr.com

PORTUGAL
Oporto
Tel: +351 22 9958698
Therapist: Ria Slof
Email: info@comodeixardefumar.com
Website: www.allencarr.com

REPUBLIC OF IRELAND
Dublin
Tel: +353 (0)1 499 9010
Therapists: Paul Melvin and Jim McCreadie
Email: info@allencarr.ie
Website: www.allencarr.com

ROMANIA
Tel: +40 (0)7321 3 8383
Therapist: Cristina Nichita
Email: raspunsuri@allencarr.ro
Website: www.allencarr.com

RUSSIA

Allen Carr's Easyway to Stop Smoking
Live Seminars & Online Video
Programme
Tel: +7 495 644 64 26
Freecall +7 (800) 250 6622
Therapist: Alexander Fomin
Email: info@allencarr.ru
Website: www.allencarr.com

Allen Carr's Easyway to Stop Drinking
Live Seminars & Online Video
Programme
Tel: +8 (800) 302 80 68
+7 985 207 47 93
Therapist: Artem Kasyanov
Email: info@allencarrlife.ru
Website: www.allencarr.com

St Petersburg
Please check website for details Website:
www.allencarr.com

SERBIA
Belgrade
Tel: +381 (0)11 308 8686
Email: office@allencarr.co.rs
Website: www.allencarr.com

SINGAPORE
Tel: +65 62241450
Therapist: Pam Oei
Email: pam@allencarr.com.sg
Website: www.allencarr.com

SLOVENIA
Tel: 00386 (0)40 77 61 77
Therapist: Grega Sever
Email: easyway@easyway.si
Website: www.allencarr.com

SOUTH AFRICA
Sessions held throughout South Africa
National Booking Line:
0861 100 200
Head Office: 15 Draper Square, Draper
St, Claremont 7708, Cape Town
Cape Town: Dr Charles Nel
Tel: +27 (0)21 851 5883
Mobile: 083 600 5555
Therapists: Dr Charles Nel,
Malcolm Robinson and Team
Email: easyway@allencarr.co.za
Website: www.allencarr.com

SOUTH KOREA
Seoul
Tel: +82 (0)70 4227 1862
Therapist: Yousung Cha
Email: master@allencarr.co.kr
Website: www.allencarr.com

SPAIN
Tel: +34 910 05 29 99
Therapist: Luis Loranca
Email: informes@AllenCarrOfficial.es
Website: www.allencarr.com

SWEDEN
Tel: +46 70 695 6850
Therapists: Nina Ljungqvist,
Renée Johansson
Email: info@easyway.se
Website: www.allencarr.com

SWITZERLAND
Sessions held throughout Switzerland
Freephone: 0800RAUCHEN
(0800/728 2436)
Tel: +41 (0)52 383 3773
Fax: +41 (0)52 383 3774
Therapists: Cyrill Argast and Team
For sessions in Suisse Romand
and Svizzera Italiana:
Tel: 0800 386 387
Email: info@allen-carr.ch
Website: www.allencarr.com

TURKEY
Sessions held throughout Turkey
Tel: +90 212 358 5307
Therapist: Emre Üstünuçar
Email: info@allencarr.com.tr
Website: www.allencarr.com

UNITED ARAB EMIRATES
Dubai and Abu Dhabi
Tel: +971 56 693 4000
Therapist: Sadek El-Assaad
Email: info@AllenCarrEasyWay.me
Website: www.allencarr.com

OTHER ALLEN CARR PUBLICATIONS

Allen Carr's revolutionary Easyway method is available in a wide variety of formats, including digitally as audiobooks and ebooks, and has been successfully applied to a broad range of subjects.

For more information about Easyway publications, please visit **shop.allencarr.com**

Your Personal Stop Drinking Plan

The Easy Way to Control Alcohol

Allen Carr's Quit Drinking Without Willpower

The Illustrated Easy Way to Stop Drinking

No More Hangovers

Allen Carr's Quit Smoking Boot Camp

The Easy Way to Quit Smoking

Your Personal Stop Smoking Plan

The Illustrated Easy Way to Stop Smoking

Finally Free!

Smoking Sucks (Parent Guide with 16 page pull-out comic)

The Little Book of Quitting Smoking

Allen Carr's Easy Way for Women to Quit Smoking

How to Be a Happy Nonsmoker

The Only Way to Stop Smoking Permanently

Stop Smoking and Quit E-cigarettes

The Easy Way to Quit Vaping

No More Ashtrays

How to Stop Your Child Smoking

The Easy Way to Mindfulness

Smart Phone Dumb Phone

Good Sugar Bad Sugar

The Easy Way to Quit Sugar

The Easy Way to Quit Emotional Eating

Allan Carr's Easy Way for Women to Lose Weight

The Easy Way to Lose Weight

No More Diets

The Easy Way to Stop Gambling

No More Gambling

No More Worrying

Get Out of Debt Now

No More Debt

The Easy Way to Enjoy Flying

No More Fear of Flying

The Easy Way to Quit Caffeine

Easyway publications are also available as **audiobooks**.
Visit **shop.allencarr.com** to find out more.

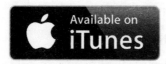 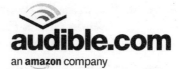

DISCOUNT VOUCHER
for
ALLEN CARR'S
EASYWAY CENTERS

**Recover the price of this book when you attend an
Allen Carr's Easyway Center
anywhere in the world!**

**Allen Carr's Easyway has a global network of stop
smoking centers where we guarantee you'll find it easy
to stop smoking or your money back.**

**The success rate based on this
unique money-back guarantee is over 90 percent.**

**Sessions addressing weight, alcohol and other
drug addictions are also available at certain centers.**

**When you book your session, mention this
voucher and you'll receive a discount of
the price of this book. Contact your nearest
center for more information on how the sessions
work and to book your appointment.**

**Details of Allen Carr's Easyway
Centers can be found at
www.allencarr.com**

This offer is not valid in conjunction with any other offer/promotion.